bunless oven

bring hope to
your trying-to-conceive tears

sandi sheehan, MA

BUNLESS OVEN

Copyright © 2013 Sandi Sheehan

Printed in the United States of America

ISBN 978-0-9848043-7-5

Edited by Lindsey Alexander
Cover illustration & design by Rejenne Pavon
Interior book design by Integrative Ink
Author photograph by Jason Wallis

Twin Petal Press
California

Contents

dedication

To my husband, Mike, who shares our life's greatest joys and our greatest losses. Who knows our pain that runs miles deep but also knew that it would someday lead us to our "hope"ily ever after. I owe everything to you and our cervical cerclage that thankfully held like steel. Thank you for working so hard for us and clearing our life's path so that I could do what I needed to do for us to get to where we are today. For encouraging me, supporting me, loving me through it all, holding my hand, being the keeper of my heart, reaching for the stars with me when it seemed we'd never reach them, and for believing we would someday make it. Guess what? We did.

To our Brecken and Caden, born one miraculous minute apart. Knowing that I would someday find my way to you offered me the ray of hope I needed to keep trying for you. Thank you for choosing me to be your mommy and for toughing it out with me for nine months of bed rest. You guys are the entire reason I made this journey. This was and is all for you. I am so blessed to be your mom. I followed my heart to get to you and I promise to always inspire you to follow your heart the same way. I love you both every minute of every day.

To our Ryan and Brayden, it is because of you that I am a mommy to your amazing brothers. You taught me how push beyond what I thought I could do and showed me how to fight without giving up. I wish I could be there watching over you, but because I can't, for reasons that are completely beyond my control, thank you for being the ones watching over me, your dad, your brothers, and Jakey dog. Even though you have gone on a step ahead of where I am, you will forever be a part of every step I ever take. I will forever love you, honor you, and blow kisses up to you and the moon.

To our baby Co. That was the name we gave you before we officially named you, because together, we formed our very own Mom & Company. It's the name that I will always remember you by. It's the blood clot that I had with you that led me to where I am today. Your passing led me to questions that later became answers, that later became preventative treatment, which ultimately led me to your brothers Brecken and Caden. You will always be my little angel.

To our very first baby, our Australian Shepherd, Jake (aka "The Dood,"), thank you for never leaving my side, for being the best bed rest buddy I could ever ask for, for licking my tears and for giving me a place to bury my head and hide when things got overwhelming, for giving me your heart to borrow while mine was broken, and for your endless patience and keeping me company with your paw and your head resting on the foot of my chair while I worked on this book. It's you who shepherded me into the most wonderful, doggy mommy-filled life. I love you beyond words. You are my hope dog.

Together, you are my seven loves, and my seven dreams come true. Thank you for showing me how to live boldly and bravely while bunless.

acknowledgements

IT IS WITH an overflowing heart that I would like to thank everyone at the Southern California Center for Reproductive Medicine for all of your dedication. Thanks to my reproductive endocrinologist, Dr. Robert Anderson, for guiding me and steering me through my infertility maze with your expertise and assurance, inspiring me to commit to my treatment path, and for kicking the butt out of every thing that ever tried to get in our way. Never does a day or milestone go by that we don't think of all of you and all you did to help us get to where we are today. To Paige Lindblad, for being such a wonderful Physician Assistant and making my care that much better. Deep gratitude to Dr. Grace Pak, for helping to restore balance to my soul with your skilled acupuncturist's hands. Heartfelt thanks to Jessica Walters, who from day one has been there for my every step backward, to the side and forward, whose uplifting spirit and heart of gold comforted me when I was most afraid. I couldn't have made it a day, or phone call, without you. Karen Smetona, my angel of a nurse, for your boundless encouragement and helping to make each cycle (and shot) the best it could possibly be. It is you who helped me to take baby steps, literally. Tori O'Cairns, for helping take the scary out of scary with our frequent office hope chats. To Robin Shapiro, who arrived to the practice not too long after I graduated on, but whose kindness has, in a short amount of time, still managed to leave a lasting impression on my heart and my boys. Sharie Parker for always keeping things running smoothly behind the scenes. And to your remarkable embryology laboratory team and the rest of your fertility care staff for helping us through the years, I am forever grateful.

To my trusted perinatologist, Dr. Marvin Posner, I will forever remember our journey together and that soft pinch on the arm that I begged you to give me the day it was actually happening for real. My hope and my wish is that you someday get to pinch every one of your patients like that. Thanks to Dr. Vivien Pan for seeing to it that my care was seamless and for lending your surgical hands during both C-sections. And to your wonderful, caring staff. Helen Nerio, for all of your kindness and for being a real source of strength to me over the years. Julie Canoy, for being that great big blue sky beyond the storm clouds. Lynne Majidian, Carla Moreira, Kathy Taylor, Tiffany Ulrich, and Sandy Pinzon, for rooting us on and being such supportive cheerleaders.

My eternal thanks to RESOLVE, the National Infertility Association, for all of the work you do to improve the lives of those affected by infertility. Thank you for bringing such hope to my life. You, my friends, are the reason I never felt alone.

Special thanks to the Twin-to-Twin Transfusion Syndrome Foundation, and founder Mary Slaman-Forsythe, for giving me the strength and resources I needed to get through a twin pregnancy all over again and actually make it to the finish this time. From one TTTS mommy to another, it's an honor to be part of your promise kept.

To all of my fellow bunless oveners, our shared stories of trying to become pregnant (or stay pregnant) connect us to each other in the deepest of all ways. May my hope find your hope and make yours even stronger.

To my entire family, my hope started with you. Thank you for all of your love and for showing me early on how to take leaps, follow my dreams, and how to get back up after a fall. Without you, I wouldn't know how to be the mom that I am.

Erin Martin, my very first fertility-challenged friend, I can barely contain the appreciation that I hold in my heart for all of the unwavering support you have given me. Thank you for being there every step of the way, and for giving me my first real glimpse of hope and IVF dreams come true with first your Kai and later your Drew. You're such a blessing.

Michelle Lether, for staying with me, holding my hand, and taking time away from your precious kiddos to help me fight for mine.

Anne Faust, our angel of a labor and delivery nurse, who personally sacrificed to be there for us on the worst day and the best day of our lives, almost two years to the day apart.

Pastor Rich Anderson, for dropping everything to be there for me in my greatest time of need, and for helping me rest my hope again on the wings of ladybugs.

Kari Wyatt, for being the kind of best friend that is usually only found in fairy tales. I am so lucky to have you in my life.

Marianne Welding, for sharing your own heartache and Heaven with me.

Donna D'albert, my treasured friend, who was the first to visit me in my bedroom hideout after my world came crashing down. Thank you for sitting with me when it hurt to breathe and for helping me lift my head up again toward the stars.

Desi Boller, for being the sister that I never had but always wanted.

Tiffany Jorgensen and Greg Yutani, for being Jake's other doggy parents during my nine months of bed rest. Thank you for the incredible gift of your friendship.

Brayden Bockler, one of the most amazing eight-year-olds I know, for all that you have done for my family. I could have never made it through to my hope and healing without you.

Teaz, the beloved Australian Shepherd who passed away before I had the chance to meet you, for the mark you and your lost litter of puppies have forever left on my heart and family.

Thanks to Lindsey Alexander, my editor, for your thoughtful edits and encouragement.

Thanks also to Rejenne Pavon, my book cover designer, for helping to bring the cover of my dreams to life.

And last but not least, to Olga Grlic, who told me there's no need to acknowledge you. I wanted to at least include you in some small way because if I hadn't, it would be like the stars not being able to thank their sky or the ocean not being able to recognize their sand—it's just unimaginable to me. You are the most magical mentor that anyone could ever wish for (and actually get).

"baby-making" defined

I'D LIKE TO share my definition of "baby-making" with you, so that we can both be on the same hopeful page.

Prior to my infertility, my definition of baby-making was defined by overflowing optimism. Baby-making, to me, meant that I would be able to conceive a baby or babies of my own, without help, and without facing any problems whatsoever. In my early baby-making days, my definition of baby-making was somewhat narrow. During that time, I didn't know anything different. I thought that things were going to be simple.

When my unexplained infertility diagnosis was first determined, the overwhelming impact of the words "You have infertility" caused me to feel that, as a baby-maker, I was broken. It was hard for me to feel hopeful about my baby-making future. I started to feel helpless about how my baby-making was going to be from that point on.

Since a cure for my unexplained infertility wasn't possible, but treatment was, my idea of what it would take to "baby-make" transformed to fit my new trying-to-conceive reality. During this time, my definition of baby-making became much more complex. Even so, it was now open to all of the various possibilities still in front of me. It moved with me in between cycles, through Clomid, intrauterine insemination (IUI), and even in vitro fertilization (IVF), something that I never thought my baby-making definition would, but later did, include.

Throughout my journey, my definition of baby-making has adapted, changed, and grown. At one point in my journey, my definition of baby-making nearly drowned in grief, retracted into a tiny ball, and I experienced, through loss, the deepest suffering that my belly and I had ever known. It took some time, and a lot of tears, but my definition of baby-making eventually became being strong enough to keep trying to conceive. Fortunately, and in many ways miraculously, my baby-making efforts paid off and my definition of baby-making came full circle, returning me to the hopeful place I started. I finally became a mother.

I've always known that, for some, the hope of conceiving a biological child is unfortunately dim. In this case, my definition of baby-making hope is not meant to give any false reassurances. After years of failed treatment, one of my closest friends was told that she probably would not be able to conceive a child of her own. That isn't to say that she and I don't still talk about her baby-making, because we do. It just means that when we talk, our definition of baby-making is bigger because we focus on other baby-making hopes—finding a donor, choosing a surrogate, or even adopting a child.

So, what I am saying is that my definition of baby-making doesn't just mean the ability to become pregnant naturally and have a biological baby. Rather, it is all-inclusive. It reflects all of the ways we bunless oveners build our families and make it to our hopeful ever afters.

introduction

I REMEMBER THE days before I knew all that was possible. I was scared. I was alone. I felt lost in this great big world of other people's pregnancy glows and blinding-in-size baby bumps. I spent most nights crying myself to sleep and praying that my infertility circumstances would change. No matter how hard I tried for a belly-to-be of my own, my stomach remained stubbornly flat. Well, bloated really. Bloated from my infertility meds, but at the same time flat.

I was thirty-five when I began my trying-to-conceive journey, so you'd think that I'd be jumping for joy that my stomach was on the flatter, fit side, but I wasn't. Ever since I can remember, all I ever wanted to be was a mom. To me, my belly was a sign that I was getting baby-making nowhere, and on most days it made me tearful to even look at it. On the outside, to most people, I am sure I came across as relatively composed, but on the inside I was punching myself, pounding the ground, and trying with all of my might to pull my very own miracle from the storks in the sky. Yet there were no pregnancy test sticks with BFPs (big fat positives), and no bun in my oven. There was only a deep longing to be a mother inside of my heart. I couldn't believe this was how my trying-to-conceive was going to be. So unsure. So unnerving. So incredibly slow. It was so different from the simple story of "the birds and the bees" I grew up hearing about.

I admit, if someone had ever told me that one day I'd be trying for a baby while battling unexplained infertility, I would have said, no way. Not a chance. Not me. I was healthy. I had regular menstrual cycles. Most importantly, I had already played out my happy fairy baby tale in my mind. In the same way that in the story of Cinderella, the glass slipper is what led her to find her true love, I always expected that my belly, when I was ready for it to, would lead me straight to a baby bump. Instead, I found myself having to painfully squeeze myself into the role of an infertility patient.

I struggled with the fact that my body wasn't recognizing its own signals. It seemed all of the other ladies in the land had been invited to the mommy-to-be ball but me. I never actually lost track of my biological clock, it just took a little longer than expected for me to meet my charming prince. I was worried that life was being unjust and punishing me for waiting. I felt incredibly unlucky, out of time, and I was one of the only people in my neighborhood without a little one in a front pack or jogging stroller.

I felt a lot of sadness. More sadness than I even knew was possible. Trying to conceive was tougher than I had ever imagined it would be. At times it was almost unbearable. But, despite long stretches of heartbreak and disappointment, like a modern-day Cinderella, I held onto my hopes that dreams really can come true. I decided that I wouldn't allow my fear of possibly not being able to conceive keep me from trying. Somewhere deep within me, I knew that I had to endure all of the heel-twisting steps in front of me, if I ever wanted to make it to my hopeful ever after.

I have my hope to thank for transforming me from what I felt that I had become, (not too far from being dried up), back to the girl I once was, (still young with promise). Like a fairy godmother, my hope guided me in the most magical of ways and convinced me I was still worthy of attending the baby-maker's ball. My infertility taught me some hard but beautiful lessons. The most important one being that no matter how much my trying-to-conceive turned to rags, I didn't have to give up believing that a TTCer like me could still make it, or think that a hopeful outcome was going to expire just because my biological clock was ticking.

What started out as a few small steps turned into some pretty huge leaps. I hit the ground running, slowed to a jog, stopped, and began again—all because of hope. I went from being horrified to asking what the whole thing entailed. I went from having nothing, to miraculously having everything, to losing everything close to the finish line, to having it all again, to losing it all again, to running the race one more time when I was almost out of breath, and finally making it to the place I am today. The place where my infertility spell was finally broken.

I believe that somewhere between two baby-making extremes, the people who have it easy, and the people like us who have it hard lies the true baby-making magic. Our roads of hope. The path that helps you envision your end result despite all of your baby-making obstacles. It might be difficult for you to see yours at first, but it's there. Your path awaits you even if your baby-making has spun out of control, grown overly complicated, or come to a temporary screeching halt. The key is to show up every day, bring all that you've got, locate your hope signs one by one, and then follow them. Haven't found one yet? Just keep going until you do. These are the first baby steps to helping you and the ones you love endure your fertility struggles that right now might look and feel hopeless.

What is a hope sign, you ask? Hope signs are those little and big things that remind you that all things hopeful are still possible and within reach. Those first encouraging words you hear from your reproductive endocrinologist—"I can work with this," or "I can work with you." Those first revealing ultrasound images of your follicles, showing you that your fertility medication is working and your cycle is on track. Hope signs like these point you to the single most important hope sign of all—that infertility is not always a stamp of sealed fate. Yes, it has tagged you, and right now, you're it. But take a look around. Hopeful outcomes for baby-makers like us exist. You'll find them everywhere. Just because you begin with a bunless oven doesn't necessarily mean you will end up with one. Let that be your first hope sign.

Of course some of you are already overflowing with hope and have figured out early on that having a full tank of hope is the only way to fuel your journey and sustain you. My heart smiles for you. Your hope will take you far. My wish is that this book gives you some new ideas and tips about using hope to recharge your soul, fill your hope potholes should you hit any on your road, and to reunite your relationships if they have veered off course in any way. You are welcome here any time. The more hopefuls on board, the better. Hope is what our journeys are all about.

But, for the majority of us, navigating our less than hopeful circumstances can be unfamiliar and unsettling to say the least. Tangled up in our reproductive snags, our hope has become an event reserved only for our brighter moments, our more promising moments, like a high follicle count, a high-quality embryo, or the very thing we dream of and strive for—a positive pregnancy test. We are the ones who make a habit out of asking hope to show up and then go away. We turn hope off and on as if it were a light switch. But, in doing this, we diminish its powers, and our hope suffers as a result. It loses its momentum, and in turn so do we. If this sounds like you, don't fret. There are plenty of small steps to build up and sustain your hope again.

Then there are those of you who had your once upon a hopeful time about your fertility potential, but in your pursuit of the destination, you've lost your hope for the journey. You're not alone. You may not know us all yet, but we are out there. We felt the same way after falling down, had to pick ourselves up, try again, and eventually discovered that where we ended up was exactly where we needed to be. It's time to join us and kick the mindset that only Fertile Myrtles surround you, and that you will never bask in hope's sunshine.

So what keeps us from our hope? Without a doubt, those of us faced with difficulties getting pregnant often interpret our fertility struggles according to a narrative that we are somehow broken, inadequate, or incomplete. For some of us, this tale becomes so strong that it prevents us from interpreting our baby-making any other way. Without a roadmap, we mistakenly believe that the mere presence of our infertility issues or our partner's issues means that our circumstances are inescapable. Most of us do not realize just how powerful our infertility stories really are. In fact, they are often so powerful that they have brute force to completely write off hopeful possibilities. We tell ourselves nothing can be done, and we begin to believe that. Where does this leave us? Mostly, running in circles, feeling that nothing will ever be better.

It's not surprising that so many of us, when trying to make sense of our complex fertility problems, screech through our so-called flashing red lights, racing recklessly to the finish line in anticipation of our happily ever never afters. We spend all of our time looking at what's gone wrong and how we are going to fix it. But in attempting to find answers to our biggest and most pressing questions, our repeated "What?" "Why?" and "When?" we unknowingly speed right past our hope signs and head straight for our speed bumps. We agonize over things like our age, our remaining eggs, his sperm count, his sperm motility, our et cetera, his et cetera. We falsely believe that if we can locate the root cause of our problem, everything can be fixed and be made right. But our troubleshooting efforts often backfire. That's because when it comes to fertility issues, often more than one problem exists. We fix one issue and another arises. We fix that one and up pops one more.

With so many pieces of our baby-making puzzle beyond our reach and out of our control, it's no wonder so many of us spin our wheels, get overwhelmed by all of the uncertainties, and don't know where to go. I should know. When I was diagnosed with unexplained infertility at thirty-five, my husband and I were newlyweds, and we were happily and playfully in love. Our minds were made up and both of our hearts were set on trying for a baby. But my diagnosis changed everything in an instant. While most fairy tales begin with a simple once upon a time, ours, it seemed, began with a complicated once upon a timeout. All of the baby-making confidence I started with vanished, and the tale I dreamed we'd tell was nowhere to be found.

Not knowing what to do, I did what any determined biological-clock driven baby-maker would do. I obsessed a little. Okay, I obsessed a lot. I mean, who wouldn't? I couldn't let infertility be my reality. I spent a lot of time, too long really, fighting my infertility in my head. Yet the more I tried to fix my situation, the more nothing seemed to be working. I felt defeated, and every inch of me was begging to stay hopeful. I was exhausted and filled with feelings I never even knew I had. I was convinced that I would never feel whole, and that I would feel this emptiness forever.

Without a doubt, infertility tests your every emotion. The feelings that have led you to pick up this book are feelings I have felt, lived, cried, and know. Although the steps of my journey might not resemble yours exactly, I know what it's like to be a baby-maker in limbo. Like you, infertility has been my early morning. It has been my afternoon and my in the middle of the night. It has been the tears I have swept from my cheeks when the weight of it all got to me. It has been the look on my husband's face when he first told me he was ready for us to have children. It has been the weight of my heart aching each time we received disappointing news. It has been the words that once dominated my sentences, like follies (follicles), embies (embryos), and blasts (blastocysts), as well as the words my heart has ached for and longed to hear, like, "Mommy" and "Happy Mother's Day."

It has also been a whole slew of ingredients that I never thought my trying-to-conceive would call for, like a hysterosalpingogram (HSG), four unsuccessful cycles of clomiphene citrate (Clomid), a laparoscopy and operative hysteroscopy, an office hysteroscopy (three of them), Gonal-F, Follistim, Luveris, Lupron, Cetrotide, hCG, four unsuccessful cycles of intrauterine insemination (IUI), three egg retrievals, four in vitro fertilization (IVF) cycles, two-week waits (2WW), one three-day transfer, two five-day transfers, one frozen embryo transfer of my previously frozen blastocysts, progesterone shots, estrogen patches, acupuncture, MTHFR

C677T, Lovenox, Heparin, two cervical cerclages, three different anti-contraction medications, and a whopping fifteen months of bed rest. But hey, who's been keeping track? I bet you are, too.

It wasn't until I met with my reproductive endocrinologist that I started to get a sense of my options and realized that a successful outcome was more possible than I imagined. So, rather than risk baby-making burnout, I made the decision to stop focusing on what was wrong and start looking at what was still possible.

I began imagining where hope could take me. I figured if I could locate one hope sign, I could certainly find another. I smartened up and began to reimagine the kind of baby-making world I wanted to be in. A place where I could continue trying to conceive and still feel strong and empowered despite my setbacks. A place where I could feel a rush of hope after giving each cycle my all. A place where I could look into my husband's eyes after a retrieval, reel him in close, give him a big hug and kiss and be able to say to him with enthusiasm, "Yay, we still have eggs!" A place where after each cycle, instead of being crushed beyond belief and being frustrated with my body, the words "I'm so grateful that we still have another opportunity" came to mind. A place where, even after another unsuccessful cycle, I could be fearless and have the courage to try again. A place where the title "mom-to-be" was still within reach. Hope became the most important ingredient in building up my baby-making resilience during all of the difficult times.

You don't know it yet, but there is a way to push through your infertility barricade and survive it. This holds true even if you have hit a few roadblocks, spun out, and infertility has kept you from your desired destination. Nobody said the journey doesn't also come with some long stretches of lonely road, lane changes, backing up, emergency braking, flat tires, off-roading, and road rash that can lead to some permanent scars. But infertility, undeniably, is the obstacle course that you have to maneuver if you want to survive it.

Maybe you are a newfound baby-maker standing here for the first time or maybe you've been around the baby-making block a time or two. Perhaps you've just begun to set things in motion by seeking consultation or you have just taken your first treatment step. Or perhaps things are already underway, and you are attempting your second, third, or even fourth treatment cycle. As you gain experience, trust your own sense of when you are ready to make the next step. No matter where you are on your journey or how deeply rooted in your baby-making struggles you feel, you will see that while your baby-making road may not be crash-proof, it is definitely not without hope.

Much of what I recommend might seem impossible at first. I expect that. I used to think that very same thing. But I have also seen remarkable things happen because of hope. It all comes down to making yourself a promise, a promise that you will remain hopeful no matter where your individual road takes you. When your hope comes together, it will be a breath of fresh air when you can hardly breathe, and it will keep you moving forward even if you feel frozen in your trying-to-conceive tracks.

It's true that some bunless oveners are luckier than others and aren't bunless for long. They undergo a diagnostic test or two, or start treatment, and their lives are changed in an instant. One cycle and bam! They become preggers and they're on their way. Others of us take a longer route. We're the ones who don't think twice about trudging through it all to get to our buns. From Clomid to IUI, we do it all. IVF? Sign us up for that too. Whatever we have to do, we do. We're not afraid to take on a challenge and spend days, months, even years trying to conquer it.

In these pages, it will become clear to you that your bunless oven is merely your starting point. It's what you do with it that makes all of the difference. There are many roads to resolutions, and your ability to stay hopeful is everything.

Infertility-filled baby-making can be a crazy, unpredictable weather forecast. Sometimes there are torrential rains and thunderstorms that seem like they are going to last forever. Other times there's so much fog you can't even see a foot ahead of you. It may not even look better for days, weeks, months or years. But if you hang on, there are also days with the bluest of blue skies and warm, shining sun followed by starry nights and radiant moonbeams. If you haven't had any yet, just wait and see. You will. As difficult as the conditions are, you will get through them. Each day is another day, brand new. Most importantly, ultimately, you will have your little bun or buns, no matter what road they travel to reach you.

Regardless of where you are in your journey, remember, hope—the rest will follow. By inviting hope into your bunless oven, you begin trying to conceive on the principle that all baby-making dreams can be created twice. First is the mental dream. The way you thought it would be. The second is the real picture. The story of what matters most to you, the physical dream you are actually living out day-to-day and can influence. Your baby-making can still make you feel good and inspire you despite what you're up against. It's important to believe that you are still bun worthy, because you are! Any steps you take toward hope, and every choice you make to keep it is a chance for you to discover what is possible.

You'll find that the end of the road is not always hard pavement and heartache. Many of us make it to our sweet endings and happy beginnings. I had some terrible disasters before getting it right, but I kept trying, adjusting each time, and in the process, I learned to fight back and not give up. I took wrong turns. I got lost along the way, I cried more tears in my journey than I have in my lifetime, but more importantly I found my way back. My TTC recipe improved with each attempt. I started to recognize a hope sign here, a hope sign there, and I followed them until I reached my dream destination, real live motherhood. When I finally arrived at the finish line, I didn't have a bun in the oven. I had two. I made it full circle. Twin boys.

I can't imagine where I'd be if I quit trying after my failures. Finding my hope was so much better than continuing to fight a losing battle. Remember, it is in our trying that we triumph. If I can do it, I'm fairly certain that once you get your bearings, so can you. When you realize just how strong you are, the parts of you that are right now in need of hope will be back on baby-making cloud nine in no time.

My wish is that nothing will stand in the way of the lil bun or buns you dream of. I trust that you will find the same hope I found and you will be here, too. I know you will be. When you feel your hope slipping, look for it anywhere—close family, trusted friends, here in these very pages, full of reassuring hope hugs for your worst days, your so-so ones, your joyous ones that still await you, and all of your days in between.

You've got this mama in the making no matter what road you take!

Your friend,

♡ Sandi

baby-make differently

M OSTLY YOU HEAR stories of baby-making on easy street. The place where ordinary TTCers conceive a baby with ease. You know, the glamorous stuff most people's family-building beginnings are made of. The stories people tell you about how they got pregnant after their first try, or within several months of trying but not trying. No zigs. No zags. Just a simple direct route. The same path you've always known was there and expected to take when you were ready.

Admit it, though. You're not the average baby-maker. There is no "easy" in your definition of "trying to conceive." While everyone else is getting ahead, following their simple bun-in-the-oven recipe and finding their way without even paying attention to their direction, your eyes are glued to the road. You're not one to get pregnant on the first try or by accident. With infertility on your baby-making roadmap, you have to work hard at it. And you mean business. You've tossed your basal body thermometer and fertility monitor because you're convinced that neither works the way they should. You're relying solely on a hunch, hope and hormone shots to get you to where you want to go.

Your ambitious attempts haven't paid off yet. It's hard, and you miss feeling unstoppable. Your efforts have slowed or come to a screeching halt and to say you're worried is an understatement.

You've been trying to not worry. But, it's not that simple. You're working around the clock—your biological one, of course, and you're tired of being reminded that there is only so much time to achieve all that you want to achieve.

Whether your glass is half-full or half-empty really doesn't matter to you right now, which is weird, because normally you're an optimist and you're the first to say it's full. All you seem to know is that life right now feels half-empty, half-complete and half-hopeful. Your heart was set on having a full house, but you'd be thrilled with a single swaddled little one resting in your arms. Instead, you're in a reproductive bind that you never saw coming. Your baby-making snag lies in your equipment, your partner's equipment, or somewhere in between the two. It keeps you up at night and it's frustrating you to no end.

Now that your baby-making warning light has signaled, it has become almost impossible to ignore. You can't escape the fact that things aren't quite going according to your big plan. You're scared and tearful, and understandably so. You're wrestling with a surprise infertility ingredient that others aren't, and it seems like you're constantly holding your baby-making breath. You keep telling yourself this isn't how it's supposed to be, and this isn't fair. You're right! It's not.

People have been politely pressing you left and right about your family building plans. You'd like to just once respond, "Hey, mind your own baby bump business!" You're wishing that everyone around you understood what you're going through. But you know that they don't and you're feeling alone. That's not all. You don't get to baby-make all sexy and cute, barefoot and carefree. Even your hair feels frazzled, and the only duds you're wearing these days are paper gowns in your doctor's exam room and oversized PJs on bed rest. You're headachy, hot, and simply not down with having to sport heavy baby-making combat boots into rugged baby-making terrain. You thought it would be relatively peaceful. You thought you'd look and feel beautiful. All you feel is barren.

With all that you're going through, it's easy to believe that you are the only one struggling. Your tries that haven't worked feel huge, and you probably think that this is what your trying-to-conceive will be like from now on. You might also be wondering if you'll ever escape it. Believe me when I say it's not just you. Many of us have to struggle, tackle, and tame the sometimes heart-wrenching side of baby-making before we reach our bliss. Not everything works the first time. The battle is real. The risks are big, and sometimes the rewards seem out of reach.

You're no Plain Jane.

There's nothing Plain Jane about your reproductive system, and that's all right. Mine isn't like most gals' either. For starters, I have a tipped uterus. My uterus is tilted backward instead of forward. Thankfully it didn't cause any difficulties for me. My uterus is somewhat more "high maintenance," though. While most women have benign polyps if they have any, there was nothing normal about the polyp that I had. Prior to the start of my infertility treatment, my reproductive endocrinologist removed one from my uterus that was about as atypical as they come. Because of this, my uterus is monitored and biopsied regularly by an oncologist to make sure I don't get any recurrent polyps or develop endometrial cancer (something most mamas in the making don't usually have to worry about).

I also carry the common MTHFR C677T gene mutation, but that also didn't stop me. When MTHFR isn't working as well as it usually does, it can affect our DNA and increase our risk for pregnancy complications. Knowing that I carried this gene allowed me to be proactive. When I did eventually become pregnant with the help of fertility treatment, my doctor prescribed me L-methylfolate, special B6 and B12 vitamins, baby aspirin, and daily Lovenox shots that I had to self administer that later switched to Heparin injections as my due date and scheduled C-section neared. Since being on blood thinners while pregnant carries risks for hemorrhage during and after delivery, as well as other risks for women requiring epidural anesthesia, many doctors prescribe the switch in medications. On top of all of that, I have an incompetent cervix (also known as a weakened cervix) due to surgery on my cervix when I was younger. Luckily, having a cervical cerclage during my pregnancy to keep my cervix from opening too soon helped with that, as did being on complete bed rest.

So, believe me when I say that baby-making the easy way isn't always the only way. Being a hopeful baby-maker sometimes means you've got to do it your own way. Bend here. Twist there. Take a different route. Although it's difficult to re-create the exact same kind of carefree conceiving in our bunless ovens, we can still come fairly close. Some of the most successful baby-makers there are have had to approach trying to conceive differently. I'm living proof that just because you baby-make differently doesn't mean you can't still have it all.

Throughout my journey, I've had to learn to set aside my unsuccessful trying-to-conceive attempts and adjust my expectations to fit the opportunities in front of me. Instead of insisting that I should have already gotten pregnant or that I should be getting pregnant as easily as everyone else, I focused on the fact that no one was telling me that my time had run out, or that my opportunities were no longer there, or that there was nothing left they could do. That's not to say that infertility didn't spoil the mood, because it totally did. The getting pregnant barefoot and carefree didn't happen for me. The quick timeframe—forget it. But when I dared to do my own kind of baby-making, everything changed for me. I felt stronger, more hopeful, and ahead of the game instead of always feeling like I was running behind.

Embrace the baby-maker you are.

Having fertility troubles doesn't make you less of a baby-maker, it just makes you uniquely you. Rather than trying to live up to your own idea or anyone else's idea of what a baby-maker is or should be, embrace the baby-maker you are. You, more than anyone, are showing your true baby-making colors just by picking up this book. You're showing that you're willing to work for what matters most to you. You're showing that you're willing to ask for help. You're willing to give your mind and body what it needs to do its best job for you. So while yes, you have to work harder at it than others, you are in fact still on your way.

When you embrace the baby-maker you are, you can focus on the things that really matter, like what it is going to take to get you there. It's okay to baby-make differently in a world where everyone else baby-makes the same. Your baby-making doesn't have to be anyone else's but your own.

Give yourself permission to be perfectly baby-making imperfect.

If your reproductive snag lies with you, instead of aiming to baby-make perfectly or even close to perfectly, give yourself permission to be perfectly baby-making imperfect. This doesn't mean that you should hope for the best and expect the worst to avoid being disappointed. It means that it's okay to start out with just the trying part of your trying-to-conceive and let the rest fall into place.

Most of us when starting to try for a baby expect the process to be flawless. We think "trying for a baby" means we will be only trying for a short while, but the fact of the matter is that sometimes it takes a little longer. Even if things don't feel perfect, baby-making differently doesn't mean that your trying-to-conceive days are over. It means accepting the fact that you might not get there the way everyone else does.

Recognize that you don't have the full story yet.

You certainly know how to describe what your body isn't doing, don't you? It isn't cooperating with you. It isn't responding to treatment the way you want it to. It isn't getting pregnant. It hasn't been dependable. It's time to stop focusing on all of the things that you think your body isn't doing and start focusing on all of the things that it is still capable of doing. You can do this by taking the time to realize that right now you are only seeing a small part of your baby-making story. You're probably comparing yourself to others who seem to have it all.

Having a family is not based on how easily it comes to you. The inspiring reality is that even some of the most imperfect baby-makers eventually have their little baby bundles. Know this and remind yourself of this often. You had your happily ever before infertility, and you will have your happily ever after infertility.

You are, in fact, a mom in the making, and just like anything that is in the process of being built, it takes time. There is always a bigger picture. It's not necessarily about hurry up and baby-make as fast as you can because your clock is ticking and your eggs are disappearing. It's about learning more about your body and what it's going to take to get you there. Even if your baby-making involves jumping through hoop after hoop, it doesn't have to be something for you to dread. It's about finding a way so that, even while different, it can still make you feel good and inspire you.

Instill hope in that not-so-Average Joe of yours.

If your reproductive snag lies partly with or solely with your man (if you have one), understand that for guys it's easy to feel lost in a great big male-factor infertility world. Think about it, he probably always expected that his "family jewels" would do what they needed to do when he needed them to and that Mother Nature was going to let you take care of all of the heavy-duty baby-making stuff. Knowing that the problem is with him probably isn't an easy pill for him to swallow. Feeling ineffectual, his confidence is probably lower than he's even able to communicate. Guys usually compare themselves to and want to be like other successful guys, and if he perceives that his body is failing him (and also failing you), he might currently doubt his manhood.

While your man might not have that same strong maternal urge you do, as a stand-up, take-charge kind of person (which most guys are), it's probably tough on him not having much control over your combined reproductive situation. If you've both been on the same trying-to-conceive page and have been trying for children of your

16

own, he too feels the pressure and knows that the final outcome weighs heavily on what his body can and cannot do. The best thing you can do for your man is to show him what is still possible. Just what does that mean?

All this means is that you give your guy a glimpse of what can still be. Assuming he's been seen by a physician and the physician agrees there are still chances for you both, help him see that he still has qualities that can lead to a successful outcome. Other men with male infertility factors are successful because they're willing to stick to their dreams and goals and move into an unknown future. Your job right now is to help him focus on the fact that most guys successfully scale their male-factor infertility issues and make it to the other side. There are plenty of fellas who have overcome such obstacles as poor sperm count, quality, motility, and similar issues that affect a man's ability to make things happen unassisted. Remind him that just because your baby-making process is nothing like either of you imagined it would be, that doesn't mean that you won't be able to still achieve what, right now, might seem impossible.

Make sure your partner knows that you don't need him to be a baby-making stud or superstar, that he's not to blame, and that you fully support him. If you're lost for words, mention to him that even the otherwise untouchable Superman has moments when he's naturally weakened by kryptonite, but that doesn't change the fact that he's still a superhero. Tell him, that whether it's his weak spot or yours, there are plenty of potential solutions that you can work through together as a couple. You just need him to regain some of the confidence that he once had so that you can make decisions. Stand by your man, then stand together and agree to stick to your family-building goal.

Decide that you're going to make it.

There are an infinite number of variables that affect you, both consciously and unconsciously as you try to become pregnant. Your age isn't the only factor. While your baby-making might not be going as smoothly as you hoped it would, and you might be feeling incredibly pressed for time, you have the option of refusing to see it as an obstacle.

Infertility isn't always unforgiving, even though your head might be trying to convince you otherwise because you are trying to protect yourself from being gravely let down. Here's what I say: You're already here, aren't you? You're already trying, right? You've decided you're in, right? Then you have nothing to lose by deciding right now that you're going to make it.

You might have to trade your images of getting there the fun and old-fashioned way (a romantic roll in the hay) for more of high-tech method that involves treatment, but you'll still be building a family. You'll just be doing it your own way. It might not happen overnight. It might not even happen for you this year. But your day will come. You will succeed in becoming a parent. Your future is wide open and has promise.

there's a baker in you

BABY-MAKERS ARE A lot like bakers. We're all hopefuls at heart. And as happy-go-lucky baby-makers it's only natural for us to want to rely upon and follow our simple once-upon-a-bun-in-the-oven recipes. The ones that, as little girls, we believed in. The ones that, as women, we expected we would just follow when ready. Simple. Smooth. Scheduled.

We've watched baby-making buddy after buddy achieve success without having to pay much attention to what they were doing or where they were going, we instinctively pursued the same path, expecting the same hopeful results. We give it our best attempts, only our friends seem to get there and we don't. Why? Because we have to baby-make with a surprise ingredient that they don't—infertility.

Any seasoned baker will tell you that they aren't successful in the beginning or all of the time. They often begin with one thing and end up with something entirely different. But unlike our pastry pals who keep trying no matter what kind of mess they find themselves in, when your efforts go awry, your vision crumbles. When one of their batches flops, they still ask what's possible. When one of your cycles fails, you view the world in terms of what's not. Their outlook is optimistic and overflowing with opportunities, while life the way you see it is hopelessly half-baked.

With each test run, bakers jump into challenges with both feet first, while during your failed runs you doubt your abilities. It's not that you don't believe in miracles. As an aspiring mother, you of course believe in those. It's that you don't know what to think when all that's left after each try is just you. You, and of course your bunless oven.

No baby-maker dreams of finding their way from scratch, starting over, an indefinite wait time, or an uncooperative oven. Yet somehow here you are. You've branched off from the general baby-making population into your own arena. The thought of improvising terrifies you. You've never baked without a recipe. You can't help wonder if things are ever going to happen for you.

It's easy to understand why you get discouraged and at times give up hope. But where would the world of baking be if our pastry pals gave up after their first try? There would be no mini cupcake, or tiny tartlet, or cookie crumble, or cinnamon bun, or Pop-Tart, or pastry puff, or butter roll or baby Bundt cake.

I've never met a baker who likes surprises, but bakers don't let surprises stop them. There is proof of that everywhere, and you shouldn't let your surprise ingredient stop you, either. Let's face it. Infertility by itself, without any context or resolution, can be terrifying. Terrifying because of the way that it sounds and terrifying because of what it is capable of doing. It threatens the way we know ourselves. It threatens our control over what happens next. It threatens what we as baby-makers are working so hard to achieve.

With baking come many valuable life lessons. Lessons about things like timing, patience, and endurance. Bakers teach us that things don't always go as planned and that reality often disappoints. But bakers also work through their so-called disasters, exude confidence, and have no problem putting their strengths and abilities to work. They bounce back after failures. They know that not every ingredient is always accounted for in a recipe. They maintain composure even when something in their kitchen has gone awry. They power through and they don't spend time focusing on whether or not their recipe is flawed. Instead they add a little here. Subtract a little over there. They adjust. They tweak. They trial. In some ways, just like you.

Run with what you've got.

Bakers have vision. They start with an idea of what they want and use the ingredients they have on hand. The success or failure of their efforts usually depends upon what they do with the ingredients they have in front of them. In a similar way, you've got to run with the ingredients you've got.

When it comes to your fertility potential, it's easy to fall into the trap of counting your eggs and becoming frantic if you don't think you have enough. Especially if you hear of someone having more than you have. The most important thing to remember is to use what you've got. It isn't about the friend of the friend you heard about who had twenty eggs retrieved, all of which fertilized and resulted in high-quality embryos. Nor is it about the neighbor who told you her sister got pregnant after just one simple, non-invasive, non-medicated IUI cycle. Fertility potential varies greatly from person to person. That's why it is counterproductive to compare yourself to someone else. Your journey is about you, only you, and running with the ingredients you've got.

If by chance you're one of those less than average egg producers, it makes sense that you feel there's little hope. All you can see is your low egg count. Having a low egg count doesn't mean you won't get pregnant. Just remember: all it takes is one. A close girlfriend of mine had only five eggs retrieved with one of her IVF cycles. Four fertilized. Three made it and were transferred. One took. Her first-born son, Kai, is now seven. A couple of years later, this same friend of mine, when trying for baby number two, had only one frozen embryo to work with. It was from a prior retrieval that resulted in five good embryos. Prior to that, she never had enough to freeze and store. Her single frozen embryo survived the thaw and she had it implanted. It took. Her second born son, Drew, is almost two. She calls him her little Jack Frost.

When seeing my friend with her two boys, you'd never know all of the zigs and zags that she faced while trying to conceive. Her very first IVF cycle resulted in an ectopic pregnancy. Another one of her IVF attempts resulted in a blighted ovum. A blighted ovum is a fertilized egg that implants in the uterus but doesn't develop into an embryo. Another one of her cycles was "a total bust" she called it, with only one egg retrieved. Regardless of the fact that with each cycle she didn't produce a ton of eggs, those small quantities still eventually blessed her with all that she had hoped for.

Not everyone might be so lucky with just one embryo. But never lose sight of the importance of giving each cycle all that you've got, even if it doesn't seem like much. Miracles can start with even the smallest of numbers and tiniest of things. There can still be hope even if it seems there should be no hope all.

Respect your infertility ingredients for what they can bring.

A true baker respects their ingredients for what they can bring to the table. Not for what they take away. Have you ever heard of a crustless pie, a free-form pizza, or a flourless cake? When it all comes down to it, you still have a pie, a pizza and a cake. The only difference is that the ingredients are arranged in such a way so that you get something entirely unique. Bakers may not necessarily like every ingredient they have in front of them, but they recognize that each and every one plays an important role in the final outcome. They focus on what they will eventually have, not what they eventually won't have.

Like a baker, you can respect your infertility ingredients in a similar way. You can respect your body, your body's process, and the individual way you have to TTC. It doesn't mean that you have to like what you are going through or the current state of things. It means it's okay to have some meltdown moments, but that you also recognize and honor all of the options you have available to you.

Once I started to respect my infertility ingredients for what they could bring, rather than resenting how much they were taking away, my hope improved, and so can yours.

Trying for a baby is a process, not an event.

When trying for a baby takes longer than you anticipated, it's easy to get discouraged. Like bakers, we as baby-makers are all about predictability and having everything in our baby-making life under control. We want to know that in the end our efforts will pay off and that from our ovens will emerge a beautifully risen bun, or two or possibly three (not all at once of course), but sometime soon might be nice. That's why a large number of us are planners. We're known for tailoring our family-building timeline around the ever-so-popular pregnant by age forty guideline/rule. I know I did. And like me, you probably thought that if you got any sort of jump-start on this timeline, that all would be good and that somehow your body and biology would reward you with extra baby-making brownie points sooner rather than later. That sure would be nice!

One of the toughest things about having difficulties conceiving is staying patient. Infertility delays many of our plans and leaves many of us feeling rushed. It makes us act like damsels in distress. We're waiting helplessly for our periods not to come. We're screaming if they do come. We're running from doctor appointment to doctor appointment and leaping from treatment to treatment. We're waiting for blood test results, fertility medications to work, and our partners to be off work and available. Most of the time we're pacing back and forth. We're sweating both the big stuff and little stuff, and we're usually questioning why everything we're doing isn't enough and doesn't seem to be making a difference.

Any determined baby-maker knows that the female equipment doesn't come with much of a wait feature. (Guys, your blueprints are much more forgiving in this department.) We don't do well with nature's diminishing good eggs equation. Without this control, many of us begin to feel out of time and out of hope, and we want our happily ever after to begin right now.

Even though there is that temptation to get pregnant as fast as possible because there are only so many opportunities to conceive per year, it's really important to take your time throughout your entire fertility treatment process—stimulating the eggs *and* making the baby. Patience is part of the package, and without it most of us wouldn't be able to do what we do. We wouldn't get very far.

Fertility treatment can be a very demanding process. Sometimes your day starts when everyone else is winding down or before everyone else's day begins. It takes showing up for appointments, sometimes before work or on the weekends. Other days, you might be instructed to time a trigger shot after midnight. Even when speeding through a cycle, you can only go as fast as your body will let you. It's best to do it right. Give each cycle your best and not just whatever energy is left over.

When bakers bake, they trust in the process, and when they bake their first batch of cookies, they do so with the process in mind. They don't put all of their eggs in one basket and expect that their first batch will be their best. Instead, they usually have some backup ingredients on hand because they already know that it might take another batch. Letting their experience guide them, over time they learn baking is not an event. Sometimes it's slow and they're just fine with that, because they've seen how it works and they know it's worth it.

Just because you think your baby-making has to happen on a given day or in a set month doesn't mean that it has to. While you can't control time, you are in control of the steps you decide to take. Sometimes those steps take time. It might seem like your baby-making is taking forever, but take it from a gal whose journey to motherhood took slightly over four years: forever is worth it when it all falls into place. Trust the process.

Boldly brave your unknowns.

Bakers live by being bold, taking risks, being patient, working out of their comfort zone, not making the simple things overly complicated, having self-confidence, not doubting their abilities, and going for it despite any limitations. We can learn a lot from them. They aren't afraid to experiment, nor should you be. True bakers don't let discouragement get in the way.

✴ It's time to stop feeling infertility crappy and start feeling infertility courageous! Being brave and bold while bunless doesn't mean you will no longer be scared. It means you might still be afraid of certain things, but you won't let your fears hold you back. Bolding your unknowns means finding a way to move through your fears. Moving from the secure place of what you already know to the insecure place of what you don't yet know is the only way to get ahead on this path.

Balance your elements.

Just like with baking, when it comes to infertility-filled baby-making, all things work together when balanced. Too much of one hormone or not enough of another can affect an otherwise perfectly good cycle. Not enough sleep and too much stress, and you'll run your body ragged. Lack of hope and too much worry, and your decision-making suffers.

Sometimes in the hustle and bustle of living, breathing, and sleeping infertility, we forget to enjoy the journey. It's easy to become worn out, cut down, exhausted, faded, fatigued, fed up, overworked, stressed out, disappointed, frustrated, tired, washed away, worn thin, and weathered. While there's nothing wrong with giving your infertility your full attention, it's important to balance all of your elements so that you can keep running your marathon and find some form of baby-making bliss no matter how small it is. When your baby-making is balanced, it's easier to be inspired and it's easier to have hope.

Try, try, and try again.

When bakers fail, they try again. They look beyond their failures, learn from them, and keep at it. They use the knowledge they gained from past attempts for their next go around, and so can you. When you're hopeful, you're a better problem-solver. You're better equipped to see the bigger picture. You're better able to keep going. Often times, a so-called failed cycle leads you to a successful one. At the end of the day, one thing is for certain: You'll never regret that you tried. However, you might regret it if you don't.

On the days I felt most defeated I reminded myself that I knew more than I did yesterday, and that I was farther along today than I'd been yesterday. One step closer to my dream. I didn't know how it was going to happen or how I was going to get there. I just knew that I had to get back to it and try again.

When you are trying, remember the word "trying" in the phrase "trying to conceive." At least you aren't sitting on your baby-making butt doing nothing. You are in fact trying. In life, triumphant rewards come from just that. They come from trying.

Every time you start feeling like you might not make it, remind yourself how far you have already come. If you're exhausted from your trying, agree that you've done all that you can for today, and try again tomorrow. Each new day brings new chances and opportunities. Things may appear more hopeful in the morning.

fire your fertility critic

YOU MIGHT BE regretting how much time it took you to launch your full-fledged trying-to-conceive campaign. You might also be kicking yourself for announcing to others that you have embarked on your baby-making endeavors, because you still have no baby bump to show for it. On top of that, you might be telling yourself over and over that you're now stuck, because of something that you have or haven't done. You can hardly face yourself, let alone everyone around you. You wish you had something nice to say to yourself, but right now you don't.

At times, everyone's a critic. On one hand, criticism can provide a place for airing opinions. On the other hand, it can provide a soapbox for upsetting internal conversations in which harsh things get said and hope is pushed aside. Your fertility critic is the inner critical part of you that keeps knocking yourself down over your diagnosis or failed baby-making attempts. Trying to conceive is hard enough. You don't need another someone busting your chops at every turn. Yet as kind as most of us are on a daily basis to others, we can be terribly brutal to ourselves.

There is no real way to hope yourself and hate yourself at the same time. It just doesn't work. When it comes to having baby-making trouble, it's easy to fall into the trap of blaming, criticizing, and pointing the finger at ourselves, because most of us view ourselves as the problem. We need to realize, though, that the things we say, out loud or in our minds, play a significant role in shaping our baby-making reality. The way we talk to ourselves can have real-life consequences. Our words have the power to transform the way we think about our past, act in the present, and picture our future.

I'm not saying that if you say only kind and encouraging words to yourself that your body will respond kindly in return and your struggles will be over. I wish it were that easy. My point is that words have power. They influence our thoughts. We become the words we tell ourselves. When those words aren't supportive, our hope suffers. No one benefits.

I've never met a fertility critic who was nice, even if on the outside they meant well. Most fertility critics have an unhealthy, unhelpful, and hurtful demeanor. Now why on Earth are some of us letting someone else into our personal baby-making business and letting them have any say over things? The answer is that most of us do it without even thinking about it. We unknowingly give our hope away. We sign it over to the biggest skeptic we know—our inner critic. And I wouldn't trust my inner critic to have my back. She might talk me out of hopeful avenues I might not otherwise consider. She might not even notice a hope sign, even if it smacked her arm or stuck a sticky note on her forehead.

Give your negative talk the boot.

It's hard to choose your words wisely in the heat of a baby-making crisis. But a little positive self-talk goes a long way toward helping you get you through your baby-making maze. In the same way that a person doesn't notice that they fidget when they talk or the way they repeat the word "um" until you bring it to their attention, I wasn't aware of my self-destructive self-speak until I really took time to listen to what I was telling myself during my times of greatest doubt.

Sad and anxious about my inability to become pregnant, my inner critic ran nonstop and talked quite a bit of trash. Even though I was remaining relatively upbeat on the outside, the negative nay-sayer inside of me was telling a very different story, and as with any self-critiquing pattern, I was only adding insult to already major injury—my fragile, less-than-fertile self-image.

I'm not much of a confrontational person. I see no value getting in someone's face. It seems like confrontations often become the precursor to a fight, and someone usually ends up getting hurt, which I don't enjoy. It hurts me to see others in pain. But similar to the way a sleepwalker walks in their sleep, I was blind to the fact that I was talking smack. I didn't even know I was doing it. I was confronting the infertile parts of myself in the not-so-nicest ways.

I've never been one to self-sabotage my own efforts, so at first I chalked up the notion of having an inner critic to having an unusually off day. If anything, I'm known for exuding a fairly consistent optimistic outlook, which sometimes spills over into me being overly peppy with myself. I had no idea, though, that when it came to all of my infertility stuff, I was harboring an undercurrent of negative messages. I eventually began to see a pattern that I knew I had to change if I wanted to make it to the other side. After all, people don't usually leap if they don't think they're going to make it.

Changing on the baby-making fly is never easy, but with a little cleaning house you, too, can turn your inner critic into your inner companion. Trust me, you're going to need her. The goal is to support yourself the way you might support your closest friend going through a similar situation. I would imagine if they were hurting, you would offer them your warmest and sincerest words. You certainly wouldn't be harsh. It all comes down to getting rid of your unhelpful words, and in order to challenge your words, you have to see your words coming. You've got to be able to identify your critic's critiquing patterns and when and how those patterns grab hold of you.

Do you ever see your infertility as all black or white? All good on this day or it's all bad the next? All positive or all negative with nothing in between? When you view your efforts as total failures or complete successes, the all-or-nothing pattern has sucked you in. Have you ever thought, "This cycle is a complete failure"? When you think of your baby-making in this way, it's considered a failure for the sole reason that it's not perfect. It causes you to fear any mistake you have made or any imperfections you have and to set yourself up to never measure up to your exaggerated expectations.

This way of self-communicating is unrealistic because infertility is rarely completely one way or the other. Sometimes what might be considered a bad thing to you, for example your diagnosis, can lead to what might be considered a good thing in general, like treatment.

Fertility critics often make it hard for you to see beyond your current TTC horizon. They often exaggerate the negatives and minimize the positives, putting all the emphasis on what is going wrong right now and then generalize it to other situations. They also have the tendency to get us to speak in terms of absolutes with words like "always" and "never." Words such as these take the stance that it's always this way or that something never works. If you've ever said, "This is never going to work," or "I might never be a mom," this is your fertility critic talking. Overgeneralizations like these are usually associated with a source of pain or hurt or anger. I'm sure you can recall when you were little, telling your parents, "You never let me stay up," or "We always have to go to bed early," or "I never get to play," and "You always make me come inside." When misused, not only does this type of generalizing lead to illogical conclusions, but it leads to catastrophic thinking where we view everything as all good or all bad.

If you find yourself in an endless loop of all-or-nothing beliefs, it's time to sit down and have a little chat with your inner bully. Escort her out the door and begin telling yourself different story of how sometimes bad things happen and sometimes good things happen, and that neither the good nor the bad cancels out the other. Your baby-making doesn't have to be a world of absolutes, nor does it need to be an inescapable maze. Just because something did or did not happen this time doesn't necessarily mean it will happen every time. There is still plenty of room in the middle for miracles.

Labels are for medicine bottles silly woman.

Your critic is also big on getting you to label things and call it the rock-solid truth. Ever said a word in such a way that it carried with it a sense of permanence? I know I have. I labeled myself as the problem, the infertility source, the baby-making stuck point. If you're like me and currently view yourself as the problem, then you're seeing your label as the real you. When you do this, you automatically expect little or nothing from yourself. Kind of a self-fulfilling prophecy type of thing.

Labels are counterproductive to our efforts because all of our energy goes to them instead of our potential solutions. To complicate matters, whether we naturally self-label or not, most of us have already been given an infertile label from our doctor or team of doctors. And whether it's explained or not, it's still a label that has been assigned to us.

The problem with labels when used in this way is that they often become emotionally charged and end up hitching a ride on your baby-making psyche. This only makes for more of a struggle when you attempt to get rid of that label later, because now it is a backstage pass to roam freely. Who are we kidding anyways—labels are for pill bottles!

Rather than firmly rooting your identity in your infertility, it's helpful to go with a less permanent option so that you can someday be free of it. Think of infertility as something you have to wear for awhile. Kind of like a pair of running shoes for a race, or a pair of braces for your teeth. When you remove your labels, you can see your bigger picture—your infertility's real job, which consists of helping you identify something to correct or adjust. Something to help bring back a little order to something in temporary disarray. Like providing arch support for your race or like straightening your teeth. Just because you are bunless right now doesn't mean you will never have your bun or buns-to-be.

One way to begin eliminating the labels you place on yourself is to keep a daily record of when you use them. Is it after a failed cycle? Is it when you're most tired? Is it when you see a pregnant mom-to-be walking by? Soon you'll see that there's no need to punish yourself for the infertility that you already feel so badly about.

Choose your words like they matter.

So you're realizing that you're quite the labeler yourself. So what's a gal like you to do? Not to worry, tackling your self-labels isn't as difficult as it seems. All you have to do is choose your words like they matter. Try to simply restate the same phrase using a different choice of words. For example, "I'm old" becomes "I feel old." Similarly, "I failed again" becomes "My cycle wasn't successful this go around." It just takes commitment and practice.

You can defeat your self-labels by assigning a new meaning to the label or by putting a new word in place of the label. Ask yourself, "If I could create any word to describe my situation better, what word is more fitting or hopeful?" Now write that word down. Write down a few. The goal is to take the power out of the label and rework it so that you are empowered again. It's simple: if a word doesn't work for you, drop it and replace it with one that does. Sometimes that's all it takes. Just find one word that's easier to swallow and makes you feel better about yourself and your situation.

A great way to catch yourself in the self-labeling act is to write down your deepest feelings about your infertility. It's not uncommon to not know how you sound until you really take time to look and listen. Thoughts are just as powerful as words, and sometimes they are even more powerful because thoughts are often tied to actions.

Begin by looking at what words you use to describe your infertility to yourself. Then look at what words you use to describe your infertility to others. Think of all of the words that you have said out loud maybe to your mom, your friends, your partner, yourself, also think of the thoughts you've privately held.

Here's a look at some of the things my former fertility critic used to use to say: "I'm the reason for this mess," "I'm causing our life to be on hold," "I might never be a mom," "I'm infertile," "I'm behind everyone else," "My uterus isn't cooperative," "My cervix is faulty," "My eggs are diminishing," "I took too long," "This might not happen for me," "Why did I wait so long?" "Maybe I really am too old. That's crazy to me, but maybe I am," "A real woman becomes pregnant with no problems," and "I can't believe this, I might never become pregnant."

When I paid close attention to what I was telling myself, I wasn't proud that I spoke to myself this way. I began to see that my negative self-talk was stealing my hope's spotlight. But once I became aware of my words I was able to change them, and so can you.

Firing your fertility critic isn't a one-time job. It means managing your vocabulary like your life depends on it, because it does. By soothing your self-talk, calming your internal physical reactions to your infertility, and easing your mind, you'll be able to think more clearly and stop feeling so panicked. You'll be able to keep your hope perspective.

Find your fertility flip side.

Having a positive frame of mind while facing conception hurdles can dramatically affect your TTC experience. Finding the flip side to your fertility troubles, means giving your overworked mind a rest from focusing only on your infertility. It can be as easy as replacing a negative thought with a positive one, or as simple as sprinkling a little bit of baby dust over you each morning.

If you haven't heard the term "baby dust" yet, it's what we TTCers sometimes say to each other to help keep each other's spirits up. When you send someone else baby dust, it simply means you wish that person good luck becoming pregnant. You deserve to think fertile, so there's no reason you can't sprinkle a little bit of baby dust on yourself!

Try using supportive, uplifting, positive statements from this point forward so that you can begin to get a sense of what positive messages sound and feel like. When you get used to them, they feel good. They help you go from feeling like there are only faint possibilities to seeing that there are real ones.

Here's a look at my fertility flip side: "I'm struggling with in-fertility right now, but that doesn't mean that I will be forever," "I feel broken but I'm not," "I'm doing everything I can to build my family," "I could become pregnant from my efforts. I have to keep believing in that," "I had slight endometriosis, but the doctor reassured me that he got it all. It would be helpful for me to listen to him and to let my past-tense endometriosis go," "My husband still has sperm and I still have eggs. We can still do this," "I'm not pregnant right now, but there will be other chances," "I have infer-tility, but just because I do doesn't mean that I won't get pregnant," and "It doesn't matter how long I waited, there is still time for my dream to come true."

Firing your fertility critic is one part conscious effort and the other part commitment. It's making the conscious effort to catch yourself berating yourself and committing to a non-self-loathing lifestyle, whether baby-making or not. Self-doubt is destructive. It's time to begin practicing getting into the habit of pairing yourself with supportive words and meanings to help sustain you and make the next half of your journey even more fulfilling than the first. Remember, you're not the label and diagnosis you've been given.

Just as negative self-talk can cause damage, positive self-talk can make a big impact on how you feel about yourself, increase your motivation, and help you better deal with your infertility at hand. It means making a conscious commitment to be regularly mind-ful of what your words convey, both negatively and positively, and thinking every day about how you can be the most hopeful kind of baby-maker you can be. Because without hope, most people might stop short and miss out on an opportunity. It's hard to be both positive and pessimistic at the same time. You'll see. In no time you'll ditch that label gun of yours.

Be firing firm.

Give your fertility critic an inch and she'll usually take a mile. Tell her to stop, and she'll just keep on running. Realize that it sometimes takes more than firing her once to do the trick. Don't be surprised if she refuses to go that first time you escort her out. You may not remember, but you gave her the key to your front door when you first allowed her to rule inside your head. But it's time to get it back. She's been stealing your hope, but your hope belongs to you.

By painting your baby-making as hopeless, your critic makes it hard for you to believe that things could ever be different. The truth is that things can. When she says those things to you, she's trying to protect you from being crushed, let down, and disappointed. But she's getting in the way of all that you are trying to achieve. She's setting you up for failure. You deserve better. It's time to set her free.

It's not every day your fertility critic is open and vulnerable to do what you ask. The moment is now. Fire her for good. She isn't the boss of your baby-making belief system—you are. It's time to stop being so critical. The only thing your inner voice should be telling you from this point on is, Atta girl! You can do it, and I believe in you.

stay close to your hope

I'T'S EASY TO feel hopeful when your baby-making seems to be going well and going somewhere. On the flip side, it isn't always easy to stay that way when things have seemingly slipped off track, and your baby bump still seems way off in the horizon.

When this whole not-getting-pregnant-easily thing first began for me, I still held a pretty optimistic outlook and kept a positive tone, but after the first year of trying with no results, my excitement began to dwindle. That's when I started to feel my first real discouraging feelings and disappointment. Suddenly it seemed everyone was taking an interest in when my husband and I were planning on having children.

With all of the outside pressure weighing in, my standard response of, "We're trying," was soon replaced with "We're still working on it." And every now and again, for people who really pressed me for an answer, I alternated between "Wish we had good news, but we don't yet," "It's just taking time," or "I'm going through infertility treatment right now."

The educated part of me knew that it was natural to feel disappointment following a failure, especially one experienced even in light of a well-crafted strategy. But the everyday baby-maker in me didn't care about the psychology of it all. The simple fact was that the more that people prodded, the harder it became for me to keep looking on the bright side. Not necessarily their bright side, but my own.

People would tell me not to worry. But how do you tell someone not to worry when that same someone thought that they would never have to worry in the first place? Of course I was worried. Nothing was making any sense, and having a baby was hands-down the single most important thing on my mind. I wanted to be a mom more than I could even articulate and more than my friends living out their blissful baby-making ease could ever imagine. It's not their fault they didn't know. They couldn't know. They weren't living it. Because of that, I felt very alone, and I started to see that much of the hope part of my journey would have to come from me.

Not knowing where to start, I began with putting my hope first. In front of my concerns. In front of my expectations. In front of everything else. By doing this, I was able to look after my baby-making in a way that I hadn't done before. I was able to give it the hope it so desperately needed. When I did this, I found that I was able to step in closer than my fear used to let me. I was able to plant tiny hope seeds where there used to be keep out signs. I was able to take all those parking spaces in my mind reserved for future possible letdowns and park hope there instead.

At first I had difficulty speaking in terms of "I can," and "I will." I was so accustomed to "I wish" and "If only." But with my new words came new insights and a new approach, I might not otherwise have thought of. I was able to simplify. Give myself one thing and one thing only to focus on, which was hoping my way until I got there.

Find your inner optimist.

Most of us approach our infertility as if it were a baby-making blaze. We take one look, freak out because we see flames, and take off running. You can run if you want to, but the only way to put a fire out is to face it and fight it.

Even though your trying-to-conceive feels like it's a disaster, doesn't mean that it necessarily is. The inner optimist in you would consider it to be more like controlled chaos. She would tell you that the fact you are handling things in a controlled environment overseen by your reproductive endocrinologist decreases the likelihood of things spinning totally out of control. She would also point out that there is still hope for you.

Your inner optimist helps you to take risks you wouldn't otherwise. She helps you to endure your shots. She keeps you from going stir crazy during bed rest. She helps keep you going—period. Being your own optimist is your first priority if you want to stay hopeful. Find her.

Prioritize hope.

One thing I discovered is that hope is not just a simple one-time task. It's not a commitment that you make up front and then it magically takes care of itself. Like anything important to you, it's about making it a priority. Setting up your baby-making in such a way that you are putting your hope higher on your list. Not making it an afterthought. In this case, it's about leading with your hopeful step. This doesn't mean you have to neglect everything else in life. It means that in the midst of all of your cycles, doctor's visits, shots (if you're doing them), your hope won't slip out of sight when you need it most.

See hope run.

When people ask me how I was successful in building my family, I could just rattle off a simple answer. It would be easy to say it was all because of IVF, but IVF isn't the entire story. It's what occurred pre-IVF and post-IVF and all the hoping in between that got me where I am today.

Pre-IVF I had to first make it past my fears. Beyond IVF and into the high-risk pregnancy zone, it was the same thing. I couldn't have made it through either without first visualizing myself making it. Yes, I was scared. Sometimes scared gutless. But seeing my hope in action gave me nerves of steel. What kept me hoping was a lot of mental hope imagery. It took practice. It took rehearsing how I wanted things to go in my mind.

I can recall how strongly certain images affected my mood and in turn affected my decisions. Sometimes in a positive way and other times not. When I was confident, I was more open. During my times of greatest doubt I could feel myself closing off, being afraid. I developed a thought process where I would see myself through to my future. I would have hope daydreams. I would see an action or milestone in my mind and then I would be doing it for real. I would imagine myself getting news of a positive pregnancy, having my hCG level rise, seeing my pregnancy progress, continuing my progesterone shots, seeing that yolk sac and fetal pole, hearing that heartbeat, watching my baby grow and meeting each milestone with every ultrasound, hurtling over any complications, and holding my baby in my arms. Those daydreams prepared me for the race, and made me more mentally tough.

You can accomplish this too by imagining that you are training for very own baby-making Olympics. It's about what you are doing now, even if your eventual goal is months or years away. Break things down into smaller parts: steps to take this week, next week, and the week after until you reach the place you want to be—the great win you imagine. Instead of stopwatches, weights, and speed trials, you are training with hope and working to create a picture in your mind of a successful outcome.

You aren't just seeing your hope in the distance. You're actually moving closer toward your miracle and your success. Whether you call it mental imagery, visualization, or mental rehearsal really doesn't matter. When you break it down, it is the ability to imagine all that is possible. This is a crucial tool when you are feeling paralyzed by the infertility-filled moments stacked in front of you.

You might not think you can influence your infertility, but you can. Begin every day and every baby-making task with a clear vision of making it through to the other side. Being able to picture yourself making it out of your tough trying-to-conceive complexities is an incredible motivator. The reason visual imagery helps you to stay hopeful is because you are imagining yourself making it through and doing precisely what you want. You are creating a path in your brain as if you have already walked down it. A path to follow. A path to practice on that helps you perform infertility feats simply by mentally practicing them.

Forgive any perceived missteps.

Shoulda. Coulda. Woulda. We all know them, but when it comes to staying hopeful none of them matter. Whether it's "I should have started trying sooner," "I could have been pregnant by now," or "I wish I would have done this or that," the problem with shouldas, couldas, and wouldas is the sense of regret you feel. They are standards for perfect behavior and perfect results, which don't necessarily exist in our kind of baby-making reality.

The consequence of having such rules is that you will feel like a failure every time you try to get pregnant and don't. They are only good for creating a lot of unnecessary turbulence and criticism in your life.

One way to oust these three hope enemies simply involves substituting words. For example, "I should be pregnant by now," can be replaced with "I could become pregnant from all of my efforts," or "I remain hopeful that I will become pregnant." When you redefine your shoulds, coulds, and woulds, you make them work for you, as opposed to against you.

Once you begin to realize that these terms are self-defeating, you can get rid of them for good. Don't worry if you slip up and one or two sneak out. When you notice yourself falling into the should, could, would trap, just ask yourself, "What are the advantages and disadvantages of having these rules for myself?" Do they make me happy and hopeful? Or do they just make me feel even more sad and helpless?

Look at it this way: mistakes are a natural part of life and part of the infertility journey. For me, it was more of a learn-as-I-went type of thing. For instance, I first sought fertility treatment through my former regular OB/GYN. I let her treat me for unexplained infertility with Clomid for a period of four cycles before moving on to a reproductive endocrinologist (also known as an RE). I didn't know the difference between the two. I do now. An RE is an obstetrician-gynecologist with advanced education, research, and professional skills in reproductive endocrinology.

I thought my regular OB/GYN knew what she was doing because of her repeated confident, encouraging words, "You have time." After all she had been my physician for seven years, so who was I to question her? Early in my journey I wasn't thinking of things like limitations of expertise and practice. This is the reason I never gathered information beyond the treatment protocol my former regular OB/GYN was advising. While she might have been a great doctor, she was certainly not an expert in fertility, and as time went on I learned that the expertise of general obstetrician gynecologists varies widely when it comes to infertility.

It appears now that it was in my best interest to have periodic ultrasounds to ensure that the Clomid was indeed stimulating ovulation and that the follicles were releasing the eggs. I probably shouldn't have undergone treatment with Clomid without this routine monitoring, but I didn't know that. Certainly the doctor didn't say anything to me, so I didn't know to saying anything to her. This is one of those shoulda, coulda, woulda moments that I eventually had to let go of. I found myself getting upset every time I thought about it. I kept focusing on the time I had lost instead of all of the hope that lay ahead.

Another mistake that I feel that I made almost coincided with the start of my infertility journey—the decision to shift careers and enter graduate school at the age of thirty-four. My intentions were good. I wanted to leave my job to pursue my lifelong dream career where I could have a flexible schedule and be a mom. Not only was I soon hit with our unexplained infertility diagnosis, I also had close to $100,000 in unpaid student loans. I put in long hours at all of my internships, but they were all unpaid.

My husband had to quickly pick up a ton of overtime just so we could stay afloat and keep up with our medical bills, none of which were covered by our insurance because they were infertility-related. So now here I was with no income, no explanation for my infertility, no baby, and my husband was gone the majority of the time. I was struggling. It was hard not to blame myself for playing such a huge role in all the things going awry.

Mistakes, if left unchecked, can have negative staying power. By reliving them in our mind, they can take on a voice and destructive life of their own. With regard to my Clomid treatment oversight, even long after I was in the hands of my reproductive endocrinologist I continued to beat myself up over not seeking the services of an RE sooner. But that didn't do any good. I was in the right hands, and that was all that mattered.

The best way to let go of mistakes, whether they're perceived or actual, is to turn them into lessons learned. Make the best of missteps. Bakers do it. Athletes do it too. Entrepreneurs do it. So listen up. Whatever regret you have wasn't and isn't your fault. You had no idea, did you? You made the best decision you could have with the information you had. Hopefully, you, too, are with your expert now and in the right hands. You got yourself there, maybe not the way you would have liked to, but nonetheless you got yourself there. You took a positive first step and you are no longer enduring unnecessary setbacks. It's time to forgive.

See the hope in small victories.

It's a lot easier to start with one victory rather than trying to conquer your "infertility all." When you've got baby-making work to do and the demands of your trying-to-conceive efforts seem too big to solve, the goal is to stay inspired. Sometimes that's difficult to do when you're feeling overwhelmed by the baby-making mountain in front of you.

I used to think of victory only in terms of the big victory—getting pregnant, staying pregnant, and having a healthy baby or babies in my arms. But in having such a narrow definition of victory, I was leaving out all of the little things that I had done or had been doing that were leading up to my end goal. I wasn't giving myself enough credit. So, I expanded my definition of victory to include all of the little things I had done or was doing to get there. I focused on one thing at a time and did the best that I could. This now meant pausing after a blood draw, acknowledging this small step, and reminding myself that I had just accomplished one thing to bring me closer to my dream.

When you are fixed only on your happily ever after, it keeps you from noticing what is happening right now. Instead of focusing on the huge win at the end and questioning whether you are ever going to get there, try focusing on achieving small victories. Small victories, by themselves, might seem unimportant. But a series of victories often sets hope in motion that helps you to achieve another small victory. What you are doing right now is making a difference. Small victories are what keep you on your path. Give it a try and watch how quickly you go from thinking, "I can't do that," to "I just did that."

Stay true to your baby-making steps and ignore everyone else's.

Life sometimes teaches us to base our happiness on comparisons to others. So, it's natural we'd stumble on the same approach while trying for a baby. But trying to conceive next to other doting parents and in stroller suburbia can be tough on not-yet parents. It's easy to feel left out and as if you are the only ones who don't belong on your street. I should know.

My husband and I were literally one of the only remaining childless couples on our block throughout all of our trying-to-conceive years. Although we chose our neighborhood because we felt it was a great place to raise a family, I never imagined that seeing others' daily sidewalk strolls through our front windows would take a toll on me. On certain days I went from feeling cozy and comfortable under my own roof to feeling like some sort of infertile freak. While everyone else toted his or her newborn or toddler, all I toted was my growing sadness.

The thing about planned communities these days is that they are just that—planned. Planned for families, that is, and not so much for people like you and me who have planned a ton, but whose infertility had some other plans for them first. Realizing that I, and we, didn't want to leave the neighborhood I knew I had to ignore everyone else's family path and stick to my own.

When you compare your beginning baby steps to the strides others have made, you're going to always feel like you are missing out and that your baby-making is never fair. Instead, focus on what you have to do to get to where you want, not what someone else has achieved. When you focus on your hope instead of the outcome that others have achieved, you will see there is enough hope for everyone. You can still achieve your happiness even if everyone else has already achieved theirs.

Surround yourself with other hopefuls.

It takes hope to know hope. Seek friendships with people who are like you and are where you want to be. Strike up friendships with those who make a positive influence on your hope. Surround yourself with these women. You will be able to connect, share feelings, and gain insights, and find new ways of bringing hope to your baby-making.

Even if it's a chat or text once a week. You'll be amazed what a hopeful influence other hopefuls can have on you. Sometimes, just knowing about how someone else survived and made it can be very encouraging.

Focus on the hope, not the odds.

I don't know about you, but the odds related to a women's declining fertility potential have always intimidated me. If odds are your thing and you're all about numbers, then I say get your odds on. But if you are looking to stay hopeful, you might want to consider focusing on the odds that are in your favor versus the ones that aren't. It's easy to become lost in the world of odds, but remember, even outside of the world of infertility, people are often times given odds of survival and regularly defy such odds. Odds are just odds—they need not define you.

One way to focus on the hope instead of the odds is to surround yourself with stories of success. Consider getting in touch with others just like you who have been successful. Remember, its not about comparing eggs or specifics, it's about strengthening your hope.

During a regular checkup, a friend of mine shared with her doctor that she was having wacky menstrual periods. She was having them more than once per month. It turned out she was facing premature ovarian failure, and she was only twenty-seven. The diagnosis was confirmed through blood tests and an ultrasound of her follicles.

Since there's no proven treatment to restore fertility in women with this condition, she and her boyfriend chose to pursue pregnancy by going straight to IVF because the prognosis wasn't good. Up until that point, she and her boyfriend had never tried to conceive. Now here they were, two weeks after receiving the diagnosis, suddenly starting shots and preparing for an IVF cycle. During the retrieval she overstimulated. Eighteen eggs were retrieved. Of those eighteen, they ended up with only two embryos to work with. The other embryos weren't dividing right in the dishes. So the two embryos she had were basically her (and their) only chance. Both were implanted and both took. They now have fraternal twin boys. How about those odds?

Not everyone successfully beats the odds early on. I sure didn't. Although I did become pregnant with twins after my first IVF cycle, I later ended up being hit with some of the most heart-wrenching odds of all. A pregnancy complication that occurred late in my first pregnancy that cost me everything.

With identical twins there are all sorts of events that can happen inside their placentas, but had you ever told me that I would go on to face preterm labor, preterm premature rupture of membranes, a prolapsed cord, a month-long fight in the hospital, then acute Twin-to-Twin Transfusion Syndrome (TTTS) and their passing when I was almost to the finish line, followed by a C-section infection and me becoming septic, I would not have believed you. We had already been through so much and it just didn't seem real. It wasn't because of anything genetic. Out little guys had normal chromosomes. It just ended up being a case of unsurvivable odds.

I share my odds with you not to scare you, but to demonstrate that the likelihood of something similar happening to you is literally next to none. Yes, odds do in fact exist, but you don't have to let them stand in your way of your dreams. Even though I experienced the most heartbreaking start, later, the odds turned in my favor.

Hit your hope reset button.

Luckily, hope comes with its own reset button. It can always be replenished. In the same way a plant needs light, water, and air, your hope often times needs renewing. Many people develop a hopeful outlook but forget to maintain it. Recognize when your hope needs boosting. Stop and give it that resparkle. Bring back its shine. When you take time to reset your hope, you are helping to make your hope lasting.

Love your period. Period.

Instead of getting bummed out every time your period comes, think about what your period means in your baby-making equation. You need her. You can't live without her. She means that your body is doing what it is supposed to be doing. She is the ticket to a new cycle. She stands for another chance. She means you're not in menopause, thank goodness for that. She's been trying with you, and she's working hard for you every month. So the next time your period comes, be easier on her. Hug and make up. Join forces. You might be surprised how much stronger you feel knowing she is on your side.

unveil your TTC tale

WE ALL BEGIN with our tales of trying to conceive. Our hopeful beginnings, our simple middles, and our celebratory endings. You may not tell yours often, but you know your story well. After all, you wrote it, and you carry it in the deepest depths of you.

If you're anything like me, you probably used to begin your once-upon-a-TTC tale based only on your hopes. Starting it each time with hopeful words like "I've always wanted to be a mom," and, "I have big plans for us," and, "I can't wait to hold you in my arms" as you dream of your someday baby-to-be. But all of your so-called plumbing problems may have shifted your pregnancy plot. Not that your hope has fully run out, because I'm sure it hasn't, but there are certain parts of your TTC tale that might now be highlighted with worry. If you've been trying for a while, with still no results, part of your tale might even have a hint of hopelessness to it.

If you were to skim the pages of my initial TTC tale, you would find a fairly simple story before infertility came into my life. You'd see happy-face doodles next to my suspected fertile days circled on my calendar and my basal body temperature readings scribbled in the margins. All signs that I was approaching my process in standard baby-making fashion. Back then, the only people I knew that had run into any TTC troubles were women with irregular periods, and that wasn't me, so I didn't give my fertility potential much thought. I was grateful for my consistent regular periods, and slightly overly confident, I think, because of them. Something that later proved to be in no way indicative of escaping infertility issues. But at the time what did I know?

The fact that I was under forty years of age, eager to be a mom and still had some eggs left were the only ingredients I thought I was ever going to need. It was about as simple of a story as TTC tales come: Mix ingredients together with husband enjoyably. Results will appear in weeks. Carry bun in oven for a period of nine months and dream will come true.

Little did I know that, for me, trying for a baby would be anything but simplistic. A year-and-a-half of trying with no positive results, followed by a diagnosis of unexplained infertility and then a rare uterine polyp, brought me to my next TTC chapter—despair. It was everything hope was not. It felt like a disaster and a dead end, with endless tears, treatment, and hormone-related mood swings. There were days I couldn't see beyond all of the setbacks and disappointments. My once upbeat TTC tale was now filled with BFNs, sleepless nights, growing marital tension, and financial stressors. I was discouraged. I felt powerless, and my hope was fighting to stay alive.

Each one of us has remarkably unique life experiences, all of which have conditioned us to respond to our baby-making in a particular way. Those of us with a strong desire to conceive, who are faced with difficulties getting pregnant, often interpret our fertility struggles according to a narrative that something is gravely wrong with us.

This is especially common in the case of a couple where one person learns that they are the identified snag in the baby-making process (like I did), while the other gets an "all clear" from their doctor (like my husband did.) This setup has the potential to lead to an unhealthy narrative for one or both partners. It did for me. Without my fertility fully in tact I no longer felt like a "whole woman." I felt responsible for my body's inability to become pregnant. I felt broken.

The way our TTC tale develops is determined by how we link certain events together and by the meaning we give to them. It's in our nature to try to make sense of our life's experiences, to repeat our stories to others, and to keep them alive by constantly feeding them with whatever thoughts and problems are currently in our lives. My initial story line of feeling broken is a perfect example of a healthy TTC tale turned troubled. What was supposed to begin as a memoir of my heart's high hopes, turned into a personal account of my pain and body's limitations.

Trying to get to the hope through my maze of a tale was sometimes a confusing mess. With some of my fears running the show, not only was trying to become pregnant in an undercurrent of unrealistic expectations, I had been putting an insane amount of pressure on myself to follow a predetermined path because I told myself that was the only way babies are made. I couldn't have been more wrong, but I didn't know that yet.

The way we view our TTC troubles causes us to develop certain beliefs and avoid others. Take for example, worry. Worry, by itself, isn't a bad thing. But, if you spend too much time worrying about your cycle "not going well," or "not working out," then your hope during that cycle doesn't stand much of chance. The result is that worry gets in the way, and you end up worrying about things that have yet to happen. Rather than continuing to focus on the fertility treatment you're committed to, the only story you prepare yourself for is your feared and dreaded outcome—no baby.

Why does any of this matter? It matters because when we are telling stories about our infertility, our stories can have a trance-like effect. We have the tendency to see only those things that reinforce the story we've written, and whatever is contradictory to our story goes unstoried and is unseen. With blinders on, we fail to see all of the possible paths to parenthood still out there.

Go back to your baby-making beginning.

If you want to get the most out of your hope, it helps to first take a deeper look at what your TTC tale is really made of. Your

TTC tale speaks volumes. At the root of it, is your baby-making philosophy. The way you approach your tale, think about it, live it, and tell it all influence your final chapter. You become the story that you tell yourself and relay to others around you. Tell yourself one thing and your tale has you feeling helpless. Tell yourself another and your tale includes the possibility of a hopeful ending. That doesn't mean that if you think you are will become pregnant that you will. It just means that your developing story, and the way you tell it, impacts you and affects your baby-making moves.

Where does your TTC begin? What are the most basic stories you have told yourself about how this time in your life would go? What words or descriptions come to mind when you think about your trying-to-conceive expectations? Try to respond to this memory in the most simplistic words possible. For example, "I was born to be a mom someday," or "I've always known that I wanted to be a parent."

Dig deep.

Your TTC tale is just one of the many different stories you live your life by. You have your family stories, relationship stories, and the way in which you understand your life is influenced by the larger stories of the culture in which you live. If your culture values family, it's often difficult to escape some of the social pressures to have children. For this reason, your bigger TTC picture might be tied to another's. Be sure to be on the lookout for layers. Sometimes, conflicting stories within you may exist—stories about yourself, your abilities, your struggles, your desires, and your failures. I did some of my own crazy story-making.

Look who's talking.

Next, think of the impact of your tale, as it stands right now. Who tells it? The brave side of you? The scared part of you? The part of you, who right now, is hurting? Are you quick to fill in all blanks as you nervously anticipate what's to come? Or is your story filled with patience and a hopeful kind of quiet? Is it filled with frustration because you're frustrated in your inability to make forward progress in your treatment process?

Your story might contain phrases like "I feel like I'm not getting anywhere," "I keep going around and around and nothing is happening," or "I'm not accomplishing anything but running tests." It might also include statements like, "Nothing ever works out for me," or, "This treatment cycle seems pointless."

Also, look to see if anyone else's voice has seeped in. Do you hear your partner's expectations overlapping with yours and ringing in your ear? Do your parents' expectations and concerns have their own say?

Pay close attention to whether or not you are telling your TTC tale in present tense. You might not be. Have you uncovered any similar past-tense stories about yourself? You could be finding descriptions of your life as "always being hard," "someone who was destined to battle difficult odds to make things happen," "someone who was always rushed as a kid to be on time," or as "someone who doesn't do well under pressure."

Even if some of what you find doesn't seem relevant to your TTC troubles, take note of it, because all of it matters. The way you cope with difficult situations, feeling rushed, and operating under pressure, in general, says a lot about the way you hope.

Check your story's hiding places.

In stories there is plenty of room for hiding places. Be sure to check out yours. Sometimes the story you are telling to the outside isn't the same as the story you are living on the inside. Ever told someone you were fine when you in fact weren't? I call this, "the tale of your two TTCers," because the strong part of you might be telling one story, while the scared part of you might be telling another. I was certainly guilty of that.

When I searched my story's secret places, I found that sometimes I lived two conflicting stories at once. In one story I was making strides with hope. In the other I was running in circles with heartache.

Knowing that there is more than one side to your story can help you choose which side of the story you want to be on.

Bring your fears to light.

There's no doubt about it, it's hard to be fearless in a viscous infertility fight. Infertility isn't a perceived threat it's a real one. Having babies, building a family and carrying on your genes is something you're wired to do. Infertility threatens your dreams and your expectations of what your life can be like. If fear is part of your story, don't fret. It's not wrong. It's normal.

Infertility totes with it some fairly scary stuff. But fear itself gives an incomplete picture. When you're stuck in what you fear, even if it's only for a few minutes, by default you write out some of the hope out that could otherwise be written in. What stays in and what stays out is all decided upon by you.

Allowing an incomplete picture of your future to grow strong and spin out of control has the potential to do more harm than good. Focusing on what you have failed to achieve for reasons beyond your control won't help you. It might even lead you to believe that you've run out of options. When you feel fearful, there is a built in tendency to ignore, forget, or play down memories and experiences that are contrary to the way you see the world. It's simple, if you can't see hope in all of your trying-to-conceive attempts then your hope can't see you. It's like signaling for help with no distress signal. The search crew is out looking for you, but you don't spot each other.

Before you can start focusing on all that is still possible, you first have to get beyond some of those premature and false assumptions running rampant in your head. You know, the stuff that blocks your hope. Your baby-making barricade—your infertility fears. When I dug deep into my own TTC tale, there my fears were, plain as day. There were sixteen of those nasty suckers running nonstop in my head.

My first fear was that I didn't act fast enough. I was afraid that because I waited, my chances of becoming pregnant might not be very good.

My second fear was that my only window of opportunity to become a mother might have came and went. I was filled with self-blame for not trying sooner.

My third fear was that I might not become pregnant—perhaps EVER. This fear ate me up inside, over and over.

My fourth fear was that I was responsible for holding everything up. Knowing that I was the source of the problem pained me deeply.

My fifth fear was that if I got pregnant, I might not be able to stay pregnant. Because having infertility took it's toll on my body and self-esteem, I questioned my body's ability to do anything.

My sixth fear was that all of my fertility meds might cause other problems for my health or my pregnancy down the road. I was worried about all of the potential side effects.

My seventh fear was that I might not be able to be the complete wife that I took a vow to be and that I dreamed I would be. Because my body was deceiving me, I felt that somehow I was deceiving my husband in terms of being able to build our dreams together.

My eighth fear was that I would not be able to give that most treasured part of me to my husband like I had always planned on doing. My inability to become pregnant made me feel less of a woman and less of a wife.

My ninth fear was that my husband might never hear the words, "I love you Dad" because of something having to do with me. The thought of this pierced my heart.

My tenth fear was not knowing who I would become if I didn't get to live out the Mom I felt that I was born to be.

My eleventh fear was not knowing what to do and how to live if I didn't end up pregnant.

My twelfth fear was not being able to control what was happening to me. I felt helpless over not being able to change our situation.

My thirteenth fear was that my husband and I wouldn't go back to being us or leading a normal life if I couldn't bear a child or children for us. I feared that my infertility would ruin our chances of a happy life together.

My fourteenth fear was that my husband might never be fully happy with me or our marriage if I couldn't bear a child or children for us. I was afraid that my husband would not fully be able to accept or love me because of my infertility.

My fifteenth fear was that my husband would resent me for not being able to give him his dream.

And lastly, my sixteenth fear was the biggest, scariest, deepest, most painful fear I kept hidden and never spoke of to anyone. I told it only to my journal. The fear that my husband would realize that he couldn't bear to live as part of a family without children and leave me to find someone else to build a life with and have children with and become a family without me because I wasn't able to give that to him.

What are some of your biggest TTC fears? Perhaps you're afraid it will be something you will not be able to give your partner, or perhaps you have the fear of being unfulfilled because you've always wanted children, or maybe you're afraid you're not really a parent if you don't reach biological parenthood. It doesn't matter if you happen upon any fears, it matters what you do with them. It's the same thing as thinking you can't do something versus thinking you can. When you know what you're afraid of, you can begin conquering your fears and pulling yourself away from all of the pain they cause you.

Find your voice.

Somewhere underneath everyone else's expectations of you is your own voice—our own TTC calling. It's what fuels your desire to build a family and keeps you committed to your path. Learning to separate yourself from the story everyone else has for you can make all of the difference as to whether or not you take a helpless baby-making road or a hopeful one.

There is always space between the stories you tell yourself and the results you want. Sometimes the way we view our infertility and the stories we tell about it becomes one of our biggest baby-making obstacles. Our baby-making minds are capable of misperceptions, some of which have the power to keep us from moving forward. It's about letting go of what you thought your baby-making was going to be like, and focusing on what it still can be like.

There are real strengths in you that you may not see in yourself yet. It's time to affirm that voice of yours that allows you to realize your full baby-making potential and get back to your hope happy place.

brighten your baby-making story

You DIDN'T COME all this way for your story to be that you have infertility, you are stuck here waiting, a family is not possible, and it's over. Well, I guess you could run with that version, but I know you don't fully believe that, and inside that's not what you want. If your baby-making story has felt more hopeless than hopeful at times, it's okay. It's never too late to let your hope back in. If you're open minded, you can begin to see your story with brand-new eyes. Find that hopeful baby-making blue sky of yours again. And tell a new story now.

Your story is your captured expression and experience, and your outlook on life. When you tell it, you're saying, "This is who I am," "This is what I am about," and "This is what I am capable of." Whether it's big and robust or small and simple, your story is a replica of how you see yourself. It's something that you will take with you, and that will serve you for the rest of your life. Think of it like your own baby-making fingerprint. It's there, making an impression, even if your infertility is opposing you.

Believe in what you're doing.
The bright side of baby-making becomes possible when you live not the story you have previously told or been told but the story

you are wanting to live. Some might call this overly hopeful. I just call it a necessary mindset in order to beat infertility. How can you build a family if you don't believe you are destined to succeed? For example, the story "I'm infertile" is filled wounds, failure, and perhaps has a tragic ending. In contrast, the story "I'm a fighter against infertility," is filled with determination and possibilities for success.

Having told your story in this way is way of standing up to your infertility and making an impact on it, rather than allowing it to just steam-roll right over you. This helps you live out your hope to the fullest in this moment.

My TTC tale took on new shape and direction when I started to break all my own rules and rewrite some things in order to counteract the incomplete truths I had been telling myself. It began with acknowledging the fact that sometimes things in life don't happen the way you think they will, but that doesn't mean that they won't happen. Every time a fear snuck in, I reminded myself that just because I was facing such a rough start didn't mean that I would have a rough finish. It also began with taking away the self-blame.

Make your infertility something you have, not something you are.

If you blame some part of yourself or all of yourself for your infertility, it's time for a relationship change. The problem is not you. The problem is your relationship to your infertility itself. Infertility is something you have. You are not your infertility, though your mind might not always be understanding or forgiving of that fact.

Now that you have seen the effects of your infertility on your TTC tale, come to know how it operates and works in your life, the next time it gets you down you can change things up. You can choose to revise your relationship with it, or even end your heartbreaking relationship with it. That's right, you can break up. Split. Dump your infertility so that your infertility is not who you are as a person.

By making your infertility an external influence in your story, rather than a trait or characteristic of yourself, your infertility doesn't get to be the leading character, you do. When you create some space between you and your infertility, you can better connect with your intentions and find new grounds for your hope. It's how your solutions come to the forefront and how your infertility moves to the background. From here, you take control of your own destiny. You'll be able to regain the hope you started with, restory your infertility on your own terms, and reauthor all of the possibilities in your TTC tale.

Go ahead, ditch the word.

There is no doubt about it, whoever came up with the word "infertility" is kind of a moron. No disrespect, of course. It really isn't a big enough word to incorporate any sort of hope. Wouldn't you agree? The "in" part of the word, acts also like an "un." "Un" words have a permanence about them. The word "infertile" sounds so carved in stone, and infertility is anything but that. Though you'd never know any sort of hope just by looking at the word.

While the medical communities use the term to reference those who are not able to get pregnant after at least one year of trying to conceive, or for at least six months if they're thirty-five or older, some non-medical dictionaries still associate the word with not being capable of producing offspring, or better yet, with being sterile or barren. Hmm, where's the hope in that? Even the phrase "temporary insanity" sounds hopeful. It's right there in the meaning. It's temporary.

Why can't infertility be called something like "temporary reproductive challenge"? I'd even settle for something like "acute female reproductive disorder." Even political candidates running for president, who might not even stand a chance at winning, are still referred to as "presidential hopefuls." Why can't we be "parent-to-be hopefuls"? When we ditch the word and find our own identity in the face of our infertility, we can be as hopeful as we want to be.

At the time of my diagnosis, I really didn't know what the word "infertility" meant. To me it had an escapable ring to it, and it didn't sound good. My mind jumped to all sorts of conclusions thinking about the worst-case scenario, and my fear got the best of me as I became trapped in and fixated on the word. It didn't take longer than a few minutes and I panicked. I thought that having infertility meant that I'd never be able to have children. It actually made me mad, too, because all a long the OB/GYN that I had been seeing for years kept telling me I had time. Now suddenly she was saying I didn't. I had so many questions. For starters, why wasn't she saying that I had a problem with fertility instead of labeling me as infertile if she actually didn't know for sure?

Looking back I'd have to say that my head-on collision with my diagnosis terminology was my first moment of infertility feistiness. Part of me didn't give a flip who was saying what about me. I was determined to escape the confines of the word. I didn't think about nicknaming my infertility. It just sort of happened. I wanted to call my uterus and my so-called infertile parts something else. Something that had more hope built into it. Something that wasn't so depressing. Something that allowed me to be temporarily affected by it. Something for a baby-maker in limbo, not a baby-maker in it's-never-going-to-happen land. That's where the phrase "bunless oven" came in. I've always dreamed of having "a bun in the oven," so this was my way of saying right now I don't have one, but I very well might someday.

From there it just sort of stuck. A bunless oven is still open. It still holds a space. It still has opportunity, and just because a bun wasn't in it didn't mean there wouldn't be one later. In ditching the word "infertile," I felt stronger. Instead of identifying with a seemingly empty word, I could focus on an oven that could still be filled.

I'm not saying you should deny your infertility nor am I advocating that you hide from it. I certainly didn't. I'm just saying that if you are going to have to live with it for a while, you might as well take some of your power back and name it what you want.

Referring to it as "infertility" gets old and depressing after awhile. Who wants to tell or live the same old story over and over again for that matter? Plus you might as well get a head start. People who are pregnant have all kinds of nicknames for their embryos.

Names like "lima bean," "little monkey," and "peanut." They don't walk around calling it "my fetus." Probably because it allows them to bond and it gives them hope.

If nothing else, you can ditch the word infertility and come up with your own code word. It's time to break free of your baby-making chains and claim your own identity.

Find one up side in your upside-down cake.

If anyone had ever stopped me along the way and told me that there was a possible upside to my infertility journey, I of course would have fought them over the notion. I couldn't see how there could be any sort of upside to my infertility when it seemed like such a wrecking ball. I initially struggled at the thought of giving infertility any credit for bringing anything good into my life, but when I took a closer look, I realized that with it came a few very distinct and beautiful gifts. I'll go first. Then you try.

The first gift I received during my infertility journey was one of the biggest, although I certainly didn't view it as a gift at the time. I can honestly say that having infertility might have actually contributed to saving my life. As part of my infertility evaluation, I underwent a hysterosalipingogram (HSG), an X-ray of the uterus and fallopian tubes. This is a commonly prescribed initial diagnostic test to help a physician evaluate the condition of the uterus and function of the fallopian tubes. During this test my uterine cavity filled normally when the contrast material was injected and my fallopian tubes appeared to be normal. However, it was concluded by the radiologist that there was a possible uterine mass they called a uterine leiomyoma.

After the test, I asked for my HSG images. I went in with just my purse in hand and came out holding a huge envelope with scary pictures. As if I didn't have enough already going on. I now had this scary possible uterine leiomyoma on my mind. A uterine leiomyoma is a tumor found in the wall of the uterus. Another medical term for it is a fibroid. Almost always, fibroids are not cancerous, but nonetheless it was still a tumor, and tumors, benign or not, still scared me.

The very next day I made a follow-up appointment with my regular OB/GYN. During my appointment I asked her to go over the radiology report with me. She seemed fairly nonchalant, told me not to worry, and said that most likely it was some sort of fibroid, which many women get. She said she wasn't concerned about it, but that if I wanted her to, she could order an ultrasound. She said there was no rush. Oh, there was a rush, I thought. I explained to her how much I wanted to conceive a baby and stressed the importance of getting to the bottom of things if in fact the fibroid would need to be removed. I asked her if an ultrasound could be ordered right away. She agreed and put in an authorization for one.

About a month later I had a pelvic ultrasound. The results came back and the radiology report concluded that no fibroids were seen. Although my OB/GYN at the time seemed satisfied and pleased with results, I still found them somewhat unsettling. I couldn't help but be suspicious. How could one report show one thing I thought while another showed something entirely different? Rather than take any chances, it was at this moment that I decided to part with my OB/GYN and move on to a more aggressive physician, a specialist—a reproductive endocrinologist, to get a second opinion.

During my very first consultation and evaluation with my reproductive endocrinologist, he performed an ultrasound right there and then in his office and located the so-called uterine mass. He diagnosed it as a uterine polyp and recommended that it be removed. Uterine abnormalities, such as endometrial polyps, can lead to lower implantation and pregnancy rates. This to me was a sign that I did the right thing by trusting my instincts and leaving my OB/GYN and getting another opinion. I didn't want surgery, but I trusted his recommendation because I wanted to get pregnant more than anything. If having this polyp out would maximize my chances for success, I was all for it. And just like that, the surgery was set.

During my laparoscopy, my reproductive endocrinologist removed the polyp as well as some mild endometriosis that was present on the surface of my ovaries. The endometriosis, I didn't even know I had. But once I woke from anesthesia and my husband told me that I tolerated the surgery well and that our doctor removed the polyp and endometriosis I felt relieved.

When my pathology report came back several weeks later, it hit me like a ton of bricks. I remember I was driving when my reproductive endocrinologist phoned to give me the results. He started out by telling me that he wasn't expecting it to be anything since polyps are rarely associated with cancer, but that his assumptions were wrong. I could sense some seriousness in the tone of his voice, so I pulled over and parked so that I could safely and fully listen.

The mass that had been removed was a rare tumor classified as an atypical polypoid adenomyoma with low architecture. Suddenly I was trying to swallow this mouthful of a diagnosis. Basically this meant that if my polyp had been left untreated, it had the potential to turn into cancer down the road if the low architecture had turned to high.

Thanks to the thoroughness and diligence of my reproductive endocrinologist, this tumor was no longer there. But, even with it gone, it still carries a risk for recurrence and endometrial cancer. So to this day, I go for follow up pelvic ultrasounds, endometrial biopsies, and see my oncologist regularly to make sure I don't get any recurrent polyps. But this is a small price to pay considering the alternative.

The second gift I received prior to my infertility journey, and I carried with me during my journey. I call it the gift of Erin. She and I met through her husband. He and I used to work together at a small startup company prior to me even knowing my husband. She and I clicked from the get-go when her husband introduced us, yet we rarely got together, mostly because of our differing schedules. When we eventually did get together she shared her baby-making struggles with me. I remember sitting with her in my apartment listening to her tell her story. She cried. It made me cry, and I remember wanting to console her. Not knowing what to say, I just relayed to her what my heart was feeling at the time. I remember telling her that I had a really strong feeling that everything was going to work out for her, which it eventually did.

When I was first diagnosed with unexplained infertility, I immediately ransacked my brain trying to pinpoint anyone and everyone that I thought I would be able to confide in and relate to. I wanted to talk to someone real. I needed someone I knew had sincere heart. Erin was the first person I thought of. Even though at the time she was going through her baby-making maze I was unable to comprehend her trying-to-conceive struggles, it didn't stop her from helping me with all of her heart.

Erin became my first baby-making buddy. She taught me a lot about what to expect. She comforted me in ways that my other friends could not. And when I felt scared and clueless—and I mean really scared and clueless—I turned to her every time. And guess what? She was there. There is something special about spending time with someone who has been there, done that, and won the infertility battle. In fact it helped me in such a way that nothing else could ever compare.

Knee-deep in my own infertility mess, with my thirty-sixth birthday approaching, my husband wanted to do something nice for me, so he asked me how I wanted to celebrate. With all of our trying-to-conceive troubles weighing heavily on me, I honestly didn't feel like celebrating right then, especially since my birthday served as a painful reminder of how long I had waited to try to get pregnant, of my infertility with unknown causes, and that I was quickly approaching forty. I remember telling him that I really just wanted to spend time with Erin and her husband.

For some reason the idea of being in familiar company, since none of our other friends had a clue what we were going through, felt like the only real way to spend my birthday. This was more like a birthday wish that I shared out loud than something that I thought would actually come together and happen. Little did I know, my husband contacted them, they arranged for a baby-sitter, and they joined us for a surprise birthday dinner.

When we arrived I noticed them right away sitting at a table, and I remember that I could hardly believe my eyes. I looked at them, then at my husband, then back at them, and then back at my husband and tears filled my eyes and fell from my cheeks. It was exactly what I needed. A dose of realness, a dose of hope, a dose of Erin.

Erin and her husband were also the ones we spoke to about our upcoming IVF cycle. We had just completed our fourth unsuccessful attempt at intrauterine insemination (IUI), and we were about to set sail in uncharted waters. I was scared, uncertain, and filled with questions. It was Erin who boosted my confidence. It was Erin who helped prepare me for what to expect, and it was Erin now telling me that she had a really strong feeling that everything was going to work out for me. It was strange to be walking in her infertility shoes.

I had no idea I would ever be so blessed to have an infertility angel like Erin traveling alongside me. When I ended up in the hospital fighting preterm labor during my first pregnancy, it was Erin who snuck in quietly, sat with me, and gave me a book about how children know their mommies and daddies before they actually know them. It was Erin's frequent text messages letting me know that I was on her mind and her regularly touching base to see how everything was going that enhanced my inner strength and helped keep me moving forward.

And most importantly, I have my infertility to thank for leading me to my greatest upside, my children. This alone is why the fight is worth it. Need I say more?

Create your recipe of hope.

Now that you know what's been holding you back, you can look at what keeps you going. I call this your hope wiggle room. If you're stuck on this part and aren't sure how to proceed, sometimes it helps to think about what someone else in your life would say about your story. Or, better yet, how would someone who disagreed with your version of events tell your story? Like your doctor? Would it be the same? How would it be different and why does it matter?

It matters because when you set out to explore the possibility of multiple perspectives and different versions of the story, it helps interrupt the trance-like effect a despair-filled story can have. Sometimes, even just recognizing the dynamic of your despair can release you from its mesmerizing effect and allow you to stand outside of it. The goal is to live out, moment by moment, choice by choice, your story of hope instead.

Here's a look at my recipe before and after I gave it a hope overhaul. My yields endless salty tears became eventually yields a bundle of joy. My no bun in the oven became seeing that I had monthly opportunities for buns. My scary treatment became not so scary once I knew what it was all about. My painful shots became not as painful when I remembered to ice first. My pounds of worry, stress, and mood swings became it's okay to let myself feel. My sleepless nights became frequent hope naps. My isolation from others, marriage difficulties, financial hardship, and seemingly dead end road, became being in the company of my fellow baby-making buds, keeping my wingman close, having a financial plan, and a hopeful horizon. When I did this, it was easier to see that I was still trying and still trucking and every day I was doing the best that I could.

Reflecting on situations that you previously overcame will remind you that you can be brave and strong again. Recall your courage, examine your resistance, and look back to the times when you weren't hopeless about a seemingly hopeless situation. Commend yourself for getting through that time in your life. Summons that strength you exhibited, that resilience, that patience, or whatever it was that helped you through that time, and know that it can be yours once again. All you have to do is copy your moves. When you feel your hope slipping, remember that feeling of strength and reenact that role. It's time for you to write your own hopeily ever after.

vent some steam

IF YOU'RE ANYTHING like me, you probably spend a lot of energy reacting to the way your infertility makes you feel. You can't help it. Everywhere you look something about your infertility wounds you or triggers you. Perhaps it's the thought "Everyone else is getting pregnant but me," or the feeling "I'm sad that my embies aren't implanting or that my hormone levels aren't what they should be." Or the frustration—"I'm tired of all of this waiting." Or the building anger—"I hate the fact that nothing seems to be working." Or the fear—"I'm scared that I won't be able to conceive."

Even though you're all for thinking positively and you try not to let you're your TTC troubles get in the way of your baby-making sunrise, they still do. You want to view each day with hopeful eyes, and you can do it successfully for a day or two. But no matter how hard you try, you can't seem to pull it off for a week, or get it to last an entire monthly cycle. Something always seems to get in the way of you trying to conceive this way.

Like any oven, even a bunless oven needs to vent steam. Venting can help you to breath easy instead of always having to breathe hard. Regulating your negative energy, if done in a healthy way, can lead you to be even more hopeful. It can help you see that even if you don't get pregnant this time, that there will be other chances.

Some psychologists today, though, will have you believe that venting to make you feel less angry is a thing of the past. They point to research that shows that hitting a pillow supposedly causes you to feel angrier. Apparently it reinforces a negative response to situations and isn't the best way to cope.

Because infertility had me go to extraordinary lengths, physically, emotionally, and financially, to get to where I am, I get a little snappish when researchers report that venting doesn't help. Let's face it. I should know a little something about whether or not some frequent offloading of infertility frustration makes you feel any better. It absolutely does. I dare you to try to convince me (or any other bunless ovener, for that matter) otherwise. No offense to my career-field colleagues.

I believe venting is a harsh reality for us TTCers. We have one of our life's biggest dreams, if not the biggest dream, on our minds, and while we are working on trying to make that dream happen some huge thing is getting in our way. Of course we are going to have a thing or two to say about it! The physical commitment alone that it took for me to make it through to the other side of my infertility resulted in more tears than I care to count. Each tear shed was a miniature vent. Crying didn't make me more frustrated. It made me less so. Occasionally ranting my frustrations didn't mean I didn't also have positive thoughts and solutions to express.

Any bunless ovener knows that sometimes you need to clear your head and offload a few worries and some negative energy, solely for the purpose of making room for more hopeful, better baby-making days.

Hope takes practice. I see a healthy batch of venting as part of that process. I'm not saying you should let yourself go on and on, venting for hours upon end, so that now there is no turning back. You can limit your vents so that you don't make a habit out of venting just to vent.

Get real with what you feel.

Since the core of our baby-making struggles threatens the way we know ourselves, most of us try to protect ourselves from the pain by moving farther away from it every chance we get. And while it may feel safer in some ways because it distances us from what hurts us most, at the same time we can also have a terrible feeling of emptiness.

While trying to conceive you are bound to have a head-on collision with everything that is running through your mind and pulling at your heart. Some feelings you might have known were there, while others might come across as a complete surprise to you. So many of us try to hold it all together, suck it up, and handle the weight of our infertility burden on our own. Others of us attempt to minimize our feelings because we don't think we are "that depressed about it," or we think, "At least I am still getting up for work everyday." On the flip side, there are those of us who overwork our infertility in our minds.

Minimization and overworking our reproductive issues are attempts by us to make sense of our infertility-filled lives. The ironic thing about feelings is that just when we think we have them mastered, that's usually when we pop. I don't know about you, but I've had my fair share of much-needed meltdowns. Hissy fits. Trying-to-conceive tantrums.

Even though I'm a little embarrassed about how I must have looked when I was storming and stomping around the house, my little outbursts helped me go from feeling stuck to being able to move again.

Where there is steam, there is also room to let it out. Whether you're sad, grouchy, cranky, or downright upset, you have a right to be all of those things. It's natural and it's important to allow yourself the opportunity and time to feel what you are feeling. When you do, not only will feel better but you'll be able to continue responding to your TTC challenges in a hopeful way. Why? Because your baby-making walls and defenses will be down.

Let it all hang out.

I've found that before true hope can be reached and help you persevere over your baby-making stumbling blocks, it's helpful to free up all the stuff that causes you the most suffering. It can be the

---

nervous energy that builds up and comes from the fru... have over the situation you find yourself. It can be the g... are doing about your body not performing the way you... expected it to.

Whatever it is, over time, your frustration, if left without a place to go, can become toxic to your hope. Remember, you're trying to make a baby. That's not something to be angry about.

I think the things that bother you most can actually help move you closer to your hopeful self once you work them out. Once you let your negative energy out you can rest and recharge in the openness that comes after all of your anger. After all of your stress. After all of your pain. In that openness is where your hope lives.

There are many ways to offload your steam. All you need now is an outlet (or several) to express yourself.

Spout it out.

If airing things out with others is something you're comfortable with, air away! Being that you might not live close to your mom or live next door to your best friend, or if you have feelings that you don't necessarily feel comfortable talking about face-to-face with someone, try funneling your feelings online. Social networking sites and the Internet make it easy to connect and share with others who have been or who are going through similar TTC experiences.

The best thing about online communities and infertility message boards is that you can give and receive support any time of day or night. You can also simply read and listen without having to contribute. It's easy to find forums that focus on general fertility and infertility issues. Forums often have separate "sub-forums" or "mini groups" for members that specifically focus on areas such as being new to TTC, endometriosis, PCOS, male factor infertility, unexplained infertility, secondary infertility, long-term infertility, infertility treatments such as Clomid, IUI, IVF, being over 35, embryo adoption and much more.

Sites like RESOLVE's Online Infertility Support Community, Fertile Thoughts, Daily Strength, and The Bump are a few of my orites. When it comes to considering medical advice of any kind, be sure to consult your own doctor to determine if it's right for your specific needs.

Put words on your worries.

Sometimes our infertility is just too much, too intense or too involved for other people to take. If you aren't up for a verbal rant or think it might frighten your loved ones away, you can always put all of your steam on paper and privately vent. When you put words on your worries, you'll come to better understand what your worries are and how they might be getting in your way of remaining hopeful.

Putting words on your worries doesn't have to be some big involved thing. It can be in the form of a simple list of all of the frustrations you feel, or all of the questions you have, or a specific worry you need to get off your chest.

It can also be a sheet of paper that includes all of the different people you have had to be during your journey so far. For instance, before infertility: temperature gauger, pee-stick monitor, calendar counter, and intercourse organizer. And during infertility: question asker, Internet researcher, appointment juggler, pincushion, shot giver, hormone producer, egg maker, sperm collector, rut-walker, penny pincher, secret keeper, blog reader, excuse maker (for getting out of numerous social events, especially baby showers), ultrasound machine hopper, tear dripper, mood shifter, and news updater.

After you've compiled your list you can tear up the pages if that helps you to get rid of more frustration.

Scribble. Jot. Journal.

So often, because trying to get pregnant was so difficult, I sometimes just sort of forgot to be present. I always found myself feeling stuck when thinking about what a struggle it all was, and how nothing about it was easy. I found it calming to have a place where I could openly offload about all that was happening in my

70

life without having to hold anything back. Even if I only s[...]
few minutes there a day, it helped.

In my journal, I could just be. I was free to express what I w[...]
thinking every single second (um, that of course, was trying to conceive) without boring or annoying the rest of the world. There was
no need to soften my speech, dance around uncomfortable feelings
or apologize for anything. I got to express all of the stuff that really
stressed me out. I got to share the feelings I felt too ashamed to
tell anyone about. I could be angry. I could be impatient. I could
be desperate. I could be sad. I could be unsettled. It was also the
place where I could hold myself together and see that I was making
progress little by little. My journal kept my hope going even if it
was nighttime, my fertility doctor's office was closed, and part of
the world was asleep.

Although my journal pages have always been written for my
eyes only, because we share similar struggles of trying to become
pregnant (or stay pregnant), I already consider you a friend. We
share stories, we share the pain, and before I can ask you to share in
the hope, I thought it might be helpful for you to see what started
me on my road from infertility frustrated to hopeful heavyweight.
Here are some of my journal entries to help you get started should
you decide you want to give journaling a try.

{sad but hopeful}

Was just diagnosed with unexplained infertility. I'm trying not to lose it, but I'm not doing a very good job. I've been bawling ever since I found out. I'm stunned that my doctor {that I've been going to forever} so casually presented this to me, especially since she's mentioned to me so many times, "Don't worry, you still have plenty of time." Without having a cause or a reason for my difficulties conceiving, how am I {and we} ever going to become pregnant? My plans for you are now backwards, sideways and upside down. None of this makes any sense. How did I {and we} get here? My hope feels all over the place. I wish I could do more to get to you. I want for you more than anything.

{haven't told you yet}

I haven't told you about my infertility yet Mom because I don't know how. You have so much going on in your own life that you don't need me to weigh you down with this right now. I don't want add to your worries you and make your life any harder than it already is. I know that when the time comes and we eventually do talk that you'll do your best try to understand, but in some ways you might not be able to understand because I'm the only one in our family who has ever had to go through this. I have no idea how I'm going to survive this. I cannot imagine not being able to have children. Being a mom is all that I've ever wanted. For now I will reach out to you in my heart, and get my hugs from you that way.

{dear best friend}

Please forgive me for keeping my infertility a secret from you, Best Friend. I'm still overwhelmed by all of this and I also don't want to rub all of this "trying for a baby" stuff in your face because, as you've have said before, at least I have my special someone. I know you sometimes think about all that I have and all that you currently don't have, and I know that's got to be hard. It's not the right time to share this with you yet, but I want you to know even though I have kept this from you I still keep you close to my heart and call upon our friendship to help me stay strong. I hope things change for me {and you, too} really soon. Love you BFF!

{counting the minutes}

My laparoscopy is next week and I never imagined that I'd need surgery to help me get to you. But here I am and here we are. I'm ready to do whatever I need to do if it means there is a chance for me to conceive you. I'm glad we now have a specialist, our RE, trying to help figure things out with us. I'm terrified of going under anesthesia though. I've never had surgery before. I told our RE that, and I appreciated his sense of humor when he replied, "Well now you have your chance." I know there are risks, but I also know that unless I keep moving forward there can be no you. I'm trying to be strong. I will continue to be strong for you. I want so much to bring you into this world. I am counting the minutes until my surgery and until you. Please wait for me.

{i wish}

My eyes hurt. My head hurts. My heart hurts. Everything hurts while I wait for you. The tears streaming down my cheeks are far too many to count. I just keep wiping them away, but they keep coming back. I'm trying for you with everything that I am. Every day without you feels like another knock down. I can't help but feel that it's my body that is failing us. I know it's not my fault. I'm still trying to accept that.

I wish it was as easy as just wanting you badly enough, trying for you hard enough, praying for you loud enough. I want to just reach up into the heavens and wrap your little fingers around mine, so that you'd at least be able to know some part of me and see how much I want to be your mom. Our lives would be so different if you were here. I just want to be your mom-to-be and decorate your nursery, but I don't want to get ahead of myself. Trying to stay patient but it's so hard.

{baby bump?}

Tomorrow is our pregnancy test. It marks the end of our third IUI. Can you believe we've done three of these? It feels like a TTC eternity! I'm really nervous. I'm also in a daze. I feel like I'm living half in our dream and half out. I have no idea what our fate is going to be. I'm worried about getting my hopes up too high like I did after our last two IUI's. It's still so crazy how both of those cycles didn't work even though our numbers and chances looked good. I don't want to keep doing this and coming up empty-handed. I've been trying to keep busy and not think about tomorrow's results but underneath it all, I'm always thinking about it. How can I not be? It's the only thing that matters to me right now. I know what's done is done, we already did what we could do, and nothing now can change things. We planted our seeds and we're either pregnant or we're not. I hope everything worked and our baby is growing inside of me. Keeping my fingers and everything crossed for us. It's going to be hard to sleep tonight. "Please let there be a baby bump!"

{aching heart}

Our pregnancy test results came back. Another big fat negative. I'm starting to wonder if this is ever going to happen for us. It feels like I'm letting everyone down, including you, someday baby of mine {and ours}. I don't have much else to say. I only have tears for today and an aching heart.

{fresh start}

It's a brand new day. My hope is back. Yesterday I couldn't do this. Today I can. I'm gathering up my strength for whatever is next. I'm grateful that my hope keeps me trying for you. Now, where were we? Oh yeah, I need to count the days until my period comes so that we can start our next cycle. I'm not letting go of my dream of being your mom. I {and we'll} find a way. Everything could change tomorrow.

Keeping a journal was another way of knowing myself. It helped quiet my mind when it was running rampant with what ifs. More than anything, it helped keep me helped keep me moving, word by word, line by line, page by page, little by little, and day by day.

Air things out together.

Most of my venting was a solo adventure, but on occasion, my husband and I found an "outlet for two" to help us with the emotional ride. On the days we vented together, it felt like riding a tandem bike. We each got to burn energy together, but also in our own, separate ways. The venting kept us moving.

After all four of our IUI's, we took trip down to the beach to mark the closing of a month-long event that we gave our very best efforts to. We both like the beach. We were married at the beach. It helped us to have a place to breathe. Each trip to the beach we would comb the sand for the largest rock we could find. Once we found one, we would lug it down to the water's edge where we would just sit with it for a few minutes. We agreed to focus all of our frustrations, disappointments, and negative thoughts onto our rock.

We brought a piece of chalk with us so we could represent those feelings in the form of words, and write them on our rock. Being the eco-conscious gal that I am, I brought the non-toxic type of chalk because I didn't want to disrupt any of our ocean creature friends when we tossed our rock into the water. When we decided we were both ready to release all that we no longer wanted to mentally and physically carry, we would signal each other. Next we tossed the rock as far out into the water as we could. This was our way of releasing our monthly heavy burdens so that we could continue along our path with as much clarity and hope as possible.

For every word we inscribed on our rock, we chose to write down on a piece of paper an opposite word representing how we saw our lives once we let go of all that was in our way, or bogging us down.

Here's a peek at one of our venting outings together. The words I wrote on my rock were: infertile, rut, sadness, problems, heaviness, debt, disappointment, resistance, pain, tears, not pregnant, without, afraid, roadblocks, empty, worry, and taking forever. The words my husband wrote on his rock were: impatient, sadness, agitation, sick, debt, without children, pain, blah, rut, dead end, separation, confusion, and closed. The words I wrote on our paper were: promise, clear path, happiness, problems resolved, inner peace, abundance, overjoyed, easier, relief, smiles, mommy, with children, brave, green lights, healthy us, together, no more worries, and complete. The words my husband wrote on our paper were: patience, happiness, calmness, health, abundance, dad, fulfilling, fun, Sandi's success, us, understanding, openness and family.

When we stopped to share our lists with each other, it was easy to see that in some ways our lists were the same and in other ways they were different. Just like the similarities and differences we faced in our journey. Venting together at the beach reminded us we were in it together. It also reminded us that we were both invested in staying hopeful, even if it meant that we sometimes held onto hope in different ways.

hope notes

ONE WAY TO keep your hopeful edge is leave yourself hope reminders. You'd be amazed how much hope you can muster up with a little help.

Give your hope little lifts.

On the days I felt my hope slipping away I left myself little hope notes to inspire myself. I stuck them on my laptop, the fridge, the shower door and the bathroom mirror. I even stuck them on my pillow. They were my hope placeholders. I call them my hope stickies. Stickies because I liked writing them on sticky notes. And hope stickies because they helped hope to stick with me. Notes like: "You can do this," "You're doing all that you can," and "You're going to get there," helped me to see that I was doing enough.

Whether it's "You're going to make it," or "Everything is going to be okay," leave yourself a little note and let it lift your hope throughout your day. Don't have any actual stickies? No problem. Many computers and smartphones come with a sticky note type of application. You can place sticky notes all over your desktop. You can also find a hopeful quote and put it on your cell phone and make it your wallpaper. You can also use your computer to "pin" little hope notes to a board on the website Pinterest. You can keep your board secret or make it public and you can invite other people to pin with you on any of your boards. A hope note can be anything you want it to be.

Don't have any hope notes of any kind just yet? Here is one from me to you: You've got this!

Visualize your hope.

Beyond inspiring yourself with pieces of paper, it's helpful to be able to picture your hope and be able to hold it in your mind. It's a vision in your head of what your life is going to be like and feel like. If not right now, then at least someday. While in the shower, I often found hope by drawing the word "hope" for myself on the steamed glass of the shower door. Most of the time I'd trace a pregnant belly. Other times I'd draw a mom holding her child's hand or have her child riding piggyback. Tracing those mommy images helped me to focus on washing my worries away, and to believe that one day that image could be me.

In addition to my water droplet notes I bought a tiny packet of self-adhesive scrapbooking design elements. One of the stickers was the word "parents." I chose that one and stuck it on a framed picture of my husband and I that I had sitting on our dresser. Every day I looked at our picture and saw the word "parents" right next to us, it helped me to really believe that someday we would be parents.

A hope note can also be something that makes you think about hope. Even a pair of socks. I wore a pair of cushy socks to every single one of my ultrasound appointments as well to all of my retrievals. It was kind of my way of putting something between me and the stirrups. Something to help me still feel like me. It's hard to feel hopeful in a paper gown. It's unnerving enough to always feel like you're on display and undressed.

My hope socks made me feel warm when I was cold and gave me my own little world of pink and blue to focus on and to hope for. They brought that little world closer to me so that I could actually visualize it within reach. They were (and still are) nothing fancy really. They are just your regular women's low-cut performance socks that are mostly white. Each pair contains a small logo on the heel and on the toe. The logo colors just happened to be light pink, baby blue, and light green. I of course dug through all of the pairs I had in the drawer and mix-matched them so that I'd have pink and blue sets. I'm sorry green socks, I had to leave you out.

To this day, I still smile and catch myself looking down at my toes when I am wearing a pair of those socks. They are still my favorite. Not because of the way they look. They are definitely worn and faded. But because of the hope they made me feel. They give me flashbacks of all those days and months I would sit with my apron draped over my lap, just waiting to see the doctor. Just dangling my toes, sporting my socks, and dreaming of the day I might be so lucky to wear them during pregnancy and be able to switch them both to pink or both to blue or one of each to represent my baby or babies-to-be.

To help me visualize my fertility, my friend Donna, a massage therapist, suggested that I place a couple of little bird nests in and around our house. Massage therapists tend to know a lot about the mind and it's role in maintaining health and wellness in the body.

I trusted her and I decided it couldn't hurt to follow her advice. I bought two nests at an arts and crafts store and put one upstairs and one downstairs. Each had its own tiny plastic eggs as hope reminders. They helped affirm the reason I was doing what I was doing and reminded me of my inner strength. I call it being a Mama Bird—the ability to watch over and have hope for my eggs. During each cycle, when I learned the number of potential follies (follicles) I had to work with within that cycle, I would put that number of eggs in each nest. And when I graduated from IUIs on to IVF, I used the nests as keepers of hope.

On my hardest days, I turned my head away from my nests for a little while. I found myself going from believing in them to being upset that they were still empty. It wasn't long though before I was back to holding them. I felt connected and drawn to them the same way I was connected and drawn to my maternal instincts. Those two little nests became part of me. They held my deepest dreams and my hope for greater fertility potential and starting a family. The nests allowed me to imagine myself as mommy without having to worry about how I was going to get there.

To this day I still have one of my hope nests by my bed. I gave the other to a friend in need of a little Mama Bird envisioning of her own. Inside of the nest are two blue eggs, a stone with the word "hope" written on it, and another stone with the word "mom" written on it.

When I found myself too afraid to decorate or buy things for the room we designated as our nursery, I focused on the two onesies that I bought and hung side by side in my nursery-closet-to-be. While at times it made me sad to look and see only two hanging in an otherwise empty closet, they brought the room and my hope to life.

Accept hope mail.

Hope notes don't have to come from you. They can come from the people you love. The people closest to you. The key, though, is to accept them fully with an open heart. Sounds simple, but it's not. Imagine yourself on your worst day. It's sometimes hard to believe you are worthy of hope notes, but you are.

I actually have my husband to thank for awakening the whole hope-note maker in me. He used to leave hope stickies for me to find. It was kind of a hope hide and seek. Sometimes I'd find his hope sticky notes in the medicine cabinet, sometimes under my pillow, always in my organizer and purse, and occasionally on the door. It almost didn't matter what the note said, once I let these little squares lift my mood, sometimes just the thought of them brought hope to my spirit and a smile to my day.

This note I found in my purse the night I attended my first peer-led RESOLVE support group meeting: "Hope you had fun and/or met some great people tonight. I admire you so much for your outlook and determination. I love you!"

During one of our tough weeks I found this note stuck to the computer screen of my laptop: "Doll, I wish I could take some of the sick feeling and pain from you and I really admire and appreciate your great way of going through all of this no-fun-ness. I am here to support you when I can and I will continue to look to how you feel to assist us in our planning for what we do or don't want to do. I love you."

Another time he stuck a sticky note on my belly. He drew a big circle to represent a hopeful embryo. Above it he wrote the words, "Any questions?"

Here are some of the other hope notes he left me. They didn't always have to do with our baby-making. He wrote them out on strips of paper: "Ahhhh! Finally a shower! Thinking of you," "All kinds of love for you," "You're my rock," and "I love you so much Cutes!"

In addition to the paper notes he would leave, his hope texts were frequent and invaluable. This worked great for my husband and I since he often works nights and long shifts. Here is a hope chat from my hubby:

My husband: One step at a time.... move a little bit more forward every day and we will realize our dreams soon enough :)

Me: Okay.

My husband: Super love to you. Don't lose sleep over things. You need that rest so that we can keep making little steps forward everyday. We'll get there.

Me: I really hope so.

My husband: Go to bed and have a restful night hiding under the covers with the Dood watching over you. It WILL pass! We'll make it. Super love.

Me: Love, right back.

And, here are two of the hope notes my mom sent me. And no it's not a typo. I call my Mom Moo. Just a little nickname I have for her. I still tear up reading them: "To Sandi, my dear daughter, I just wanted to let you know how much you are loved and you are in my heart and on my mind always. The angels are watching over you and are by your side wrapping you in their giant wings. Even though I won't be with you for your procedure I will be holding you in my thoughts. I know you will be just fine, the angels told me so. I love you so much, Hugs, Moo."

Here's the second one she sent to me: "To my lovely daughter, Sandi, know that my love embraces you even though I don't see you as often as I would like. Remember the angels will be with you throughout your journey to motherhood. I love you so much, Mom XXOO

My mother-in-law also sent me a card and wrote "hugs for when you need them" in the card. I kept it tucked in my journal. I looked at it every time I jotted down notes detailing my doctor's visits or phone conversations with our doctor.

The purpose of sharing some of my own hope notes is not to brag. Trust me, the communication between my husband and I, as well as between my Mom and I, when I was deep in the trenches of TTC, wasn't always pretty. It's to show you the power other people's words can have. It's to get you to take your own hope notes out and keep them where you can be reminded of the hope that other people have for you. During the times you aren't feeling up to hope-seeking, they can bring the hope to you. The fact is, you probably already have a hope note or text somewhere. Take the time to string your hope notes together. It will help keep your hope strong.

Build a hope playlist.

It's easy to look around you at all the sacrifices you are making and ask yourself what on Earth are you doing. Staying inspired and dedicated to your treatment path sometimes seems impossible. Sometimes you need something to put you in a hopeful state of mind or a little extra push to keep you going one more cycle. That's where hope notes in the form of music comes in. Music has a way of reigniting your confidence and often makes those sacrifices seem like they aren't sacrifices at all. That every step you take has a purpose. Having some hope tunes can do that for you.

Loading songs that carry meaning for you on your iPod or iPhone or creating your favorites list on Pandora Internet Radio, whose sole mission it is to play only music you love, might be just what you need to make it through one more injection, or through that last grueling day of your two-week wait. It's all about putting together a mix that moves you, one that will get you across your finish line. Adding and downloading songs that help you to feel strong and to stay inspired will give you that boost you need to make it through your tougher trying-to-conceive moments. Finding songs with inspiring lyrics that highlight what you want to achieve will help remind you and affirm that your dream is within your reach.

Keep in mind there are songs also out there that might really bring out your tears. Decide if a song like this would be helpful to you. For me it was. Sometimes listening to songs that allowed me to cry and feel what I was feeling helped me feel better. I made the mistake though of having my husband watch a music video that was about infertility, and it kind messed up him for the rest of the day. I think it was just too much for him. So realize that what might work for you, might not work for your partner. Be sensitive of that and give them the choice by saying, "There is a song about infertility that I listened to today that is kind of sad, but it helps me get my feelings out. Do you feel like listening to it?" That way they aren't blind-sided by something they weren't expecting.

Mostly the songs I chose weren't about infertility. They were songs about other things that made me feel hopeful. What's on your hope playlist?

If you're unsure where to start, below is a list of some of the songs that were on my hope playlist to help you start building yours.

My Hope Playlist

The Climb *by Miley Cyrus*

I Won't Give Up *by Jason Mraz*

Faith When I Fall *by Kip Moore*

Laughed Until We Cried *by Jason Aldean*

The Sun Will Rise *by Kelly Clarkson*

Little Wonders *by Rob Thomas*

Someday *by Rob Thomas*

Fix You *by Coldplay*

Somewhere Over The Rainbow *by IZ*

My Wish *by Rascal Flatts*

Stand *by Rascal Flatts*

Three Little Birds *by Bob Marley*

One Day You Will *by Lady Antebellum*

Be Ok *by Ingrid Michaelson*

A Thousand Years *by Christina Perri*

Brighter Than The Sun *by Colbie Calliat*

Here Comes The Sun *by The Beatles*

love the buns you're with

DON'T WORRY, I promise this chapter isn't about telling you that you should be satisfied with the life you currently have. It's not. It's about allowing yourself to still be in love with your life, and the loves in your life, while you're trying to conceive. It's about trying for the baby you dream of *and* loving with your whole heart the family you already have. Simply put, it's being able to count your follicles *and* your blessings at the same time.

I remember the day that I lost an enormous sense of hope and regained it all in the same day. It was a day that I was feeling more down than usual. It was a day that I was nearing my wit's end. We had been undergoing treatment for quite some time and I was having difficulty seeing beyond our current baby-making stuck point. As my husband and I stood together in our kitchen with our angel of a dog, Jake, our Australian Shepherd, at our side, the weight of it all just hit me. I instantly broke down. I remember burying my head deep into my husband's T-shirt and just sobbing there as he wrapped his arms around me. I remember crying so hard I could hardly speak. My tears were doing all of the talking for me.

When my crying reached a brief lull, my husband pulled me in even closer and whispered in my ear, "You're already a mommy, you know. You're a doggy mommy. You are his mommy," he said as he pointed to Jake. It took those few minutes, fourteen words, and one reassuring look from Jake for that message to reach the parts of me it needed to reach. My inner doggy mommy identity, the one I didn't even know I had, was now awakened, and suddenly, without really knowing why, I felt like I could breathe again.

Up until that point, I had been so focused on my idea of what being a mom was to me that anything short of my version—being pregnant—I was somewhat blind to. While nervously waiting for the beauties and joys in my life to be born, I couldn't see what being a mom was to my everyday loves. They were already seeing me as I dreamed of being, and suddenly my belief was being challenged. If I replied, no I am not, I would be denying both of them the way they saw me, and if I said, yes, I am, did I actually believe it inside?

I remember struggling with the idea of being a mom without really being a mom the way the rest of the world might define it. How can you both be a mom and not yet a mom at the same time? Little did I know that our four-legged companion would be the powerful catalyst that helped me realize I was already an exceptional mother. It didn't make up for the fact that I wasn't pregnant yet and it certainly didn't erase my pain. But it helped me focus on what I needed to focus on. In some small and big way, already being "seen" as a mom and "felt" as a mom helped me to deal with my feelings and helped me to hope even more. I had been so afraid I was never going to hear those words. I was so consumed with trying to build my future family that I was almost beginning to lose sight of the family I already had right in front of me. Of course I didn't really forget about them. But I was preoccupied to say the least.

Certainly having a loving husband and loyal pup isn't the same as having a little bun or buns-to-be, I know, but the two together made me realize that mommyhood, at least my version of it, had some definite room to grow. Room to include. Room to fill. How about yours?

Acknowledge your already mommyness.

Surely, if someone were to ask you why you think you would be a good mother, you probably would be able to answer. Do you know why? Because in some small way you already see yourself as a mother. It's completely alright for you to see yourself this way, too. It's who you are, it's what you're made of, and nothing, not even infertility, can take that away from you.

We all have mommy and daddy identities before we actually become moms and dads. If you look at a true baby-maker's core, what you'll usually find is the desire, intention, willingness, and commitment to unconditionally love your someday child or children. It's something special that we bunless oveners have. We don't take the process for granted. We're grateful for every glimpse, every possibility, every miracle. We have to work hard at it. We don't have the luxury of pregnancy oopses or by accidents. We have to walk the walk, and we miss nothing because we notice everything. But in being overly focused, we sometimes inadvertently neglect the other buns in our lives.

With Jake, I was able to acknowledge my already mommyness through our daily mommy and me interactions. Whether it was his reliance on me to feed him, his willingness for me to bathe him, his allowing me to put him in his seat belt harness when he went with me in the car, our little play dates, his trusting me to tend to his boo-boos, and letting me tuck him in at night, as a true sheepherder by nature, he managed to sheep-herd me into a doggy-mommy-filled life.

Our routine, even though it had been our routine for quite some time, had suddenly taken on a greater purpose. It was there to help turn my story around. It was there to help me hope.

My friends and family helped me with acknowledging my already mommyness, too. For as long as I can remember, my best friend Kari has always found cute little ways to honor me and recognize me as a dog and cat mommy. Same thing with my friend Donna, who once said to me, "You know, even without being a mom, you are one of the best moms I know." Every Mother's Day, she sends me this text: "Happy dog and cat mommy day." She, too, is a dog and cat mommy herself, and a wonderful one at that.

In a similar way, while I was trying to conceive, my sweet mom regularly asked me how her Granddog was, and my caring, older brother, who is a doggy dad, always made me feel as though we were deeply connected by our dogs. Aside from raising an adorable Tibetan Terrier, I'm pretty sure he thought he'd have a couple of his own kids by now, but he's currently single and still hasn't met "the one" as of yet. He's an amazing uncle to his nephews, and whenever he's around children, it's neat to see. They just can't get enough of him. He seems to have humbly moved on from his biological dreams, allowing whatever "will be" to "just be," and he's happy for all of the other things in his life. Even so, I hope he meets someone amazing (who loves dogs) and they sweep him off his feet. At least there's no biological time limit to finding love.

All of the little "mommy messages" I received reinforced to me that regardless of my bunless predicament, my closest friends, my husband, my mom and brother, my angel dog (in person) and angel cat (in spirit) already saw me as a mom. This helped me to see that I could begin living out part of my inner mom identity at every moment. You can do the same.

I'm not saying that you have to be a pet owner to experience what I'm talking about. You certainly don't. All you really need is an open mind and a handbag. What's the handbag for? So that once you realize that certain parts of being a mom are already in built into your nature, you can carry that hopeful thought and image with you wherever you go.

When you take time to acknowledge the mommy you already are, you actually free up some of your energy. Think of it as taking out a loan from your baby-making bank. You have all these re-sources within you that you have saved up. You use these resources while you baby-make. Some are physical resources, such as taking time to care for your body. Others are psychological, like psyching yourself up for a shot, or talking yourself through your anxiety about a particular treatment.

Even if you free your mind of just one of your baby-making tasks, that leaves more room for hope and more energy for investing something else into the rest of your trying-to-conceive. You get to pay yourself back with something better than something that might feel like a heavy burden. You get to pay yourself back with a hope pick-me-up.

Affirm that you are already a someday mom.

Instead of putting all of your energy into thinking about how you aren't a mother yet, when you affirm "I am a loving mother-to-be," you can baby-make while fully being present at the same time. This will make it easier to love the buns you're with. Likewise, if you are miserable and suffering and you regularly negatively affirm that you might never be a mother, and that nothing you're doing seems to be making a difference, you sometimes miss what's happening right now and you probably aren't able to give your current loved ones the best that you have to give.

Tote your natural mommy traits.

Surprisingly, once I arrived at my hopeful future, I found one small striking similarity between my infertility journey and motherhood. If someone who has never been through infertility were to ask me what infertility feels like, my answer to them would be this: It feels incredibly vulnerable. It feels like the only thing on your mind, and the only thing that matters. It feels like the hope you have and the love you have to give your someday child or children is so big, it all just sort of overflows and feels like part of your heart is living outside of yourself. On certain days it makes you question who you are. It sometimes stops you in your tracks. It gets you to look back. It gets to you to look forward. It makes you appreciate every chance you get. And if you already believe in miracles, well, it makes you believe in them even more.

The ironic part of the whole thing is that now that I've made it to other side of my infertility, if someone who hadn't become a parent yet were ever to ask me what motherhood feels like in the very beginning, my answer would be exactly the same. Of course, just minus the word "someday" before child or children. This is the reason I firmly believe that you are already toting your mommy traits before actually becoming a mom.

Love your buns, right now, with your whole heart.

Most of us know how to withdraw when we are in pain. Some of us do it even to our closest of friends. But what if this moment is all you have? Does it make sense to deprive your loved ones of your best right here and now? It's similar to the "love yourself first" principle. If you hold hope for yourself first, then you can more deeply hold hope for your future baby or babies-to-be. Why? Because your head won't be filled with negative thoughts. It will be filled with hope instead.

If this sounds difficult, it really isn't. Just begin looking for any ways that you might already be like a mom. Are you an auntie? Are you a step-mom? Do you work with children in some way? If nothing comes to mind, think about your past. Have there been any times in the past when you've been like a mom? Maybe you helped a lost boy who got separated from his dad find him again. Or maybe you donated blood and later found out that it went to a little girl who had kidney disease. Have you ever adopted an animal? Or mended a child's wound?

Obviously the idea here is not to try to replace the longing that you do have to be an actual mother in the biological sense, but rather to expand your view of what a mom is and what a mom can be, so that while you're in limbo, you can still live out a part of that role, a part of that desire, and part of yourself that you already are, without neglecting any of your current buns.

There are benefits to baby-making while fully being present at the same time. It's sometimes challenging, but it's not impossible. Loving the buns you're with has its own kind of transformational powers when you interact with your loved ones right now in whatever capacity you can. It doesn't mean you have to slow down or stop moving toward your mommy goal. It just means baby-making with your current buns at your side so that your hope can pick up momentum and act like a propeller and push you even closer to your dream.

One of the quickest ways to bring the present moment into focus is to tell yourself certain phrases aloud. Phrases like "I am here," "Right now," "Right now is all there is." Not only might this help you take that much-needed accepting sigh, it might bring you closer to the ones you love, because no matter which way you slice it, even if you have the best of intentions of always being close, when your mind is preoccupied with what it wants and your body is preoccupied with the pain it feels, it's natural to isolate yourself, intentionally or unintentionally.

When I began to see my husband as the fuel to keep me going and my Jake as my daily recharging station, I was able to include them in my infertility. With my husband, it was easier when I stopped seeing the problem as solely my own. When I did this, I made more room for his love to see me and us through, and less room for ridiculous nonsensical thoughts like maybe he didn't want to be with me if I couldn't have a baby.

My husband's job became being everything from my handy-man, to right-hand man, to my hope wingman. My dog's main role became Chief Bed Rest Buddy. He would lie at my feet when I felt like I couldn't do the infertility stuff anymore. He gave me wet nose kisses at the precise moment I needed a dose of hope. In between treatments and during our walks together, he helped me to take deep breaths. I felt he understood that we were on a mission, to rid mommy of her infertility stress. At my side, his unconditional love said everything without saying a word. Every day he stared right into my eyes as if to say, "I'm here with you, you have me and I love you, mommy."

Of course, being Jake's mom, I'm going to want to spread the news about the hope that brought to me. I think pets can be quite powerful. I believe there is something to say about the latest scientific findings on how dogs can save lives, sniff out cancer, and warn epileptics of impending seizures. Believe it or not, Jake could actually tell when I was pregnant and when I wasn't. He's quite the keen pee sniffer. Surprisingly, he was right every time. The times when my blood tests came back positive were the times he would literally put his entire head in the toilet bowl after I peed and flushed. The times when I wasn't pregnant, he acted as though he almost didn't really care if I had just peed, as if to alert me, "Sorry, there's nothing here to sniff, Mom." I'm not sure if he actually sensed my pregnancy-related hormones or what it was. He just seemed to know.

The main reason for talking so much about Jake is that when it comes to human interactions, people sometimes hesitate, hold back, and make excuses. When it comes to people-animal interactions, though, people tend to feel calmer, more relaxed, more willing to venture out, more able to let go and just be. Animals unconditionally love you and accept you no matter what your physical ailment or what's occurring around them. It's an incredible thing to experience.

If you have the opportunity, I encourage you to spend time with an animal if you can. Obviously if you're allergic to animals, a face-to-face interaction might not benefit you. However, there are other ways to interact with comforting creatures without making face-to-face contact, such as visiting an aquarium or equestrian park. You get the idea. While animals can't solve our infertility issues, they certainly have the power to soothe us and enhance our overall well-being, which goes a long baby-making way.

There will come a point in time for all of us traveling on this journey when our trials and tribulations will come to pass, but our loved ones—the buns we're with—will continue on with us long after this journey is over. And we can never get the time back once it has already passed. Your family in the making includes the family you already have. If you let them, they will love you and ride out this journey with you.

So whoever and whatever you do have, be it a partner, another child, a beloved pet, a close family member, a treasured friendship, they deserve your complete attention and appreciation for the moment being shared. Being present in the unconditional love, companionship, and support of those around you, especially when you feel as if you are at your wit's end, can be just the thing you need to invite more hope into your infertility-filled days. As you continue to wait patiently for the beauties and joys in your life to be born, you can also love the loves in your life surrounding you at this very moment. You're working toward your little one. In the meantime, you can still love now.

I wish I could say that my cat is still with me, and with us, but a couple of years ago, while I was in the hospital on bed rest for four months, she passed away. I was supposed to come home the same day she died but there was a problem with my IV pump. It broke, and my final course of antibiotics to treat the C-section infection I developed after the delivery of my boys, got delayed. If it hadn't broken, I would've gotten to say goodbye. Her passing the way she did, and when she did, still hurts. I know in my heart that once her mommy, always her mommy, but I still miss her sweet face.

Balancing being a mom and a secondary infertility patient.

If by chance you're already a mom, whose first-time baby-making efforts were a piece of cake, but you're now going through secondary infertility and you're feeling fertility-cheated the second or third time around, you too can be a hope-toting mom.

For you, "loving the buns you're with" all comes down to your ability to stay committed while you're caught between two worlds. It's making that commitment again and again to care for, and love fully, day in and day out, the child or children you do have, while trying for another. It's finding a way to balance being a dedicated parent *and* an infertility patient. That means taking care of you so that you can best take care of them.

When trying to build a bigger family when you're already raising a child or children, it's important to remember that you're in a unique situation. Having conceived a child or children without any trouble before, you might feel a great deal of pressure to conceive again, since you know it's possible to have a baby. You might also be realizing that there are no guarantees about whether or not you will go on to carry another child. For this reason, your trying for a baby isn't just between you and your partner anymore. Any TTC ups and downs you might be having can have a far-reaching impact on your entire family, even if you think your child or children might be too young to understand the complexities of what you're going through, or that they're unaffected by what you're going through because they don't see you cry.

In addition to being a mother of toddlers, I've spent several years counseling preschool and elementary school-aged children, during which time I've seen how sensitive, perceptive, and in tune with their parents young children can be. They can often sense their parents' tension, sadness, distress, or frustration. A lot of time, energy, emotions, and finances go into pursing fertility treatment or adoption. There's always that possibility that they might have overheard conversations with your partner, your doctor, or a close friend about disappointments, setbacks, or grief you're facing. Likewise, if your child has only been given the simplified explanation that "you're trying for their brother or sister," without knowing everything else you're going through, they might interpret and internalize some of those conversations (and your moods) in a negative emotional way.

The best way for you to keep loving the buns you're with is to stay attentive and engaged in your child's day-to-day activities as much as possible, continue to love them with all you've got, and proactively respond to their needs and any boo-boos while also tending to your own. It's sounds impossible, I know, but I'm surrounded by secondary infertility success stories every day. When you get the most discouraged, just keep thinking back to the hope you held for your first bun or buns. That hope can be yours again.

plant mommy seeds

ONCE MY MOMMY identity was given to me, like a gift, from my family, it instantly melted my heart and began to speak to me. It helped me to believe that I was worthy of that role, and it helped me to be a more hopeful placeholder for my baby or babies to come. I was no longer carrying the thought of me being a mom outside of myself. I was now toting it on the inside, like a tiny "mommy seed" that I couldn't see with my eyes, but that I could feel had been firmly planted and was now a part of me.

Having this first mommy seed sort of snapped everything into place, woke everything up, and helped guide my thoughts and actions. It helped me to feel more fertile. That's what mommy seeds do. They're small, hope-packed seeds, that when planted and cared for, help you to see and affirm that you're already an evolving, beautiful mom in the making.

Advocates of affirmations believe that what we most often tell ourselves can become reality. I used affirmations all throughout my infertility to help restore my faith in my own body and point my focus toward a happy future. Each one helped keep my hopeful mindset going.

By planting mommy seeds, you're choosing to be bold and deliberate with your intentions. You're affirming that you're worthy of a mommy title and a wonderful life as a mommy. Then you're stepping back and letting go so that they have time to grow and blossom from your vision into something real. This is an important step, because sometimes what grows is so much better than what you dreamed up.

If you want to come up with some mommy seed affirmations of your own, but you're running into difficulty coming up with any, try to think about the way you would speak to your best friend if she were facing difficulties trying to conceive. What would you say to her? Now try telling those same things to the person who needs to hear them the most—you.

Here are some of the affirmations I affirmed to myself. Feel free to use any or all of these, or write your own: "My bunless oven is open and ready," "My fertility treatment is moving forward every day," "My mind is open to this working out," "My babies are waiting patiently for me," "My cycle is going strong," "My body is receiving the help it needs, and it knows how to do its job," "My belly is beautiful even if it's plumped full of meds," "I know that I will beat my infertility," "I will get pregnant this year," "I am already a mom-to-be," "I am already a mom in the making," "I am the perfect age to be a parent," "I am a hopeful about my baby-making," "I am baby-making the best I can every single day," and "I know that pregnancy will happen at the right time for me."

The beauty of mommy seeds is that once they are planted they continue to grow and change, just like you will continue to do throughout your journey. When I finally became pregnant, my mommy seeds grew into supportive pregnancy affirmations. After all that it took to finally get to that point, I knew I was going to need some heavy-duty hope to see me through all of my worries. So I wrote things down like, I will hear my babies' heartbeats, my pregnancy is strong and resilient, and I will meet my healthy babies on their due date. My mommy seeds helped me to stay calm.

So now it's your turn to plant some mommy seeds, invite hope in and watch your very own mommy seeds grow.

hope times two

I RECENTLY MET a gal who has chosen to fly infertility treatment solo, without a partner, and all I can say is she wowed me. I can imagine just about anything on this journey, but I can't imagine venturing it alone. Thankfully, most of us have our significant other also going through this with us. But even if you don't, your "hope times two" can be anyone you want it to be.

The saying that love conquers all is a saying I gravitate to and actually believe in. But when it comes to trying to balance battling infertility and your relationship, I think a saying more like, "love and hope" conquers all is actually more spot-on. Sometimes even a great relationship can be thrown for a loop by when you literally have to fight for a baby. Heads can disagree. Directions can change. Hope can clash. When it does, it sometimes makes it hard to be on the same hopeful page. Coordinating hope is no easy task, but I think couples can and deserve to be hopeful no matter what they are facing.

Crisis has a way of building closeness or creating problems in couples. Moodiness often becomes moodiness doubled. A small spat often turns into a heated argument. Everything seems to come and go in cycles, including hope. Sometimes it's hard enough just trying to scrounge up enough hope for you, let alone find a way to hold onto enough hope for two.

When my husband and I first began our baby-making, our hope was contagious. As newlyweds, we had it in our heads that our baby-making forecast would be filled with crystal-clear blue skies, and we had no reason to believe it would be otherwise. Instead, it dumped rain for several years, at times hailed, and even snowed us in a few times. Some days our hope was frozen. On our worst days we spent many of our nights together bickering, spooning only occasionally for warmth.

During times of higher stress, our home was often a baby-making war zone. Both of us just trying to survive in our own separate ways. We had so much "infertility" fight in the two of us that at times we would find ourselves strong-arming each other instead of fighting our fight the way we wanted to, hand-in-hand and side-by-side.

My husband was caring, but at the same time he was clueless, (through no fault of his own of course.) He wasn't the one with the infertility issues, I was. It wasn't that he wasn't supportive. He was. It was that often he was supportive at the wrong time or in the wrong way. It was difficult for him to show empathy and compassion for something he, himself, had never gone through.

Surely, he didn't mean to be dismissive of my feelings, but at times he was. He also didn't understand that certain social settings were painful for me. He repeatedly misinterpreted my, "I'm not in the social mood right now," as me "hardly ever wanting to go out with friends." He didn't get the fact that while some get-togethers were enjoyable for him, because he had other guys to talk light-hearted sports talk with, that those same backyard barbeques were agonizing for me because of all the gals talking about pregnancies and babies.

Other times he thought that I was just being overly sensitive, when in fact, I had every reason to lose it and have tears pouring down my cheeks. I carried the weight of my body being our hold up, not him. So in many ways he didn't "get it" or "get me." Your partner might be clueless about some of these same things too.

In our case, my husband not actually having the infertility made it difficult for him to help me and for us to be able to relate on most days. We had different concerns weighing on our minds, and he was way less physically involved the process than I had to be. That alone created a great divide, and at times I wished our roles could have been reversed. We tried and we tried real hard, but our wants, realities, and hormones didn't always match up. It wasn't just that our stars weren't lining up—we as a baby-making couple weren't aligned. We were out of hope harmony.

It took us awhile, but we finally learned to administer emergency marriage first aid, build a shelter, and signal for help when we needed each other. In the end, he wasn't oblivious. He got better at supporting me with practice. With enough TLC, our frozen hope eventually thawed just in time for another treatment cycle. With each cycle we improved.

The two of us definitely learned how to hope together the hard way. But we did learn. We learned that in order to survive in our climatic baby-making extremes, we had to join forces and use our natural gifts to come through our situation. His natural gift: his strength. My natural gift: my hope.

We also learned that a successful partnership goes beyond appreciation for each other, which we had, to preparedness and cohesiveness, which we lacked. We adopted a more easy-going style with each other, and that was when our hope clicked into place. Me allowing him to hope his way, and him allowing me to mine. Of course, we still had our moments, like occasionally when one of us would hide or bury our hope out of fear of being disappointed. But little by little we learned how to avoid stepping on each other's hope toes so that we could invite hope to stay.

If your twosome could use a little hope boost of its own, here are a few ideas that will help you to hope your way together.

Connect in some small way, every day.

Relationships carry added stress if they don't keep their connection going. It only takes a few minutes to touch base. Both carrying demanding jobs? Not to worry. Touch base before or after an appointment, a meeting or a task you are carrying out for the day. Most of us aren't full-time baby-makers and have other life commitments to balance in addition to our treatment.

Taking time to check in with your significant other isn't as difficult and time consuming as you might think, and it goes a long way. Say hello to texts. I was never a huge texter, but my husband's texts to me quickly became my trusted hope lifeline. There were several times he was not able to go to my appointments with me. His texts were like hope notes in my pocket. With all the uncertainty surrounding our future, I knew I could at least always count on his texts to tell me he was with me every step of the way. Even if you aren't big on public displays of affection, just squeeze hands really quick. It's like having your own hope handshake saying psst, I am still here.

Have each other's baby-making back.

Someone needs to have your back, why not the two of you? Never underestimate the value of your partner even if he isn't the one with the infertility diagnosis. Yes, there can sometimes be huge gaps in understanding and empathy between you if you are the one with the primary diagnosis, but don't lose sight of the fact that you are going to need each other to get through this. It's just as much his problem as it is your problem. Why? Because whether you like it or not, you are in this together. You are a team. You are partners.

There are small, simple things you and your significant other can do every day to help each other. It can be rough in the baby-making trenches when you are dodging fertility landmines, financial pressures, and time crunches, not to mention sometimes other people's uninvited comments about your baby-making plans. If all else fails and you both need to feel supported, say this to each other as often as you need to, "Love, I've got your back."

Forgive disagreements and agree to hope.

Sometimes disagreements happen. One of you might be working long hours and the other of you is braving all of the meds. One of you might be on bed rest while the other is handling all of the household chores. Tensions might be high. Frustration might be overflowing.

Trying for a baby through infertility can be hard. It takes its toll on you both. When and if you find yourself in a disagreement, agree to disagree about the disagreement. Know that you both mean well. Then agree to hope. Neither one of you necessarily has to hope the same, but you have to at least both agree to invite it into your thoughts, your hearts, and your baby-making.

When you overhaul the way you look at your disagreements, and choose to forgive your misunderstandings, it changes the way you interact. It lets you be both be human. It allows you both to have bad days. And while you might temporarily diverge in your conversation, when you forgive and agree to hope, you come back together. Agreeing to disagree is not always comfortable, and sometimes it means letting go of your pride. But when you do you, it will allow you both to focus on what is most important.

Believe me when I say there are a few head-butting moments my husband and I shared in the midst of our roughest times that I still remember clearly, of course. But I was able to forgive them and look at them almost as though they happened to other people. When we agreed to disagree about everything else but agreed on hope, we were able to focus on the things that really mattered to us and forget all of the rest. We are living proof that you don't have be a perfect couple to be a hopeful one. Over time our disagreements transformed us for the better by building the skills we needed to truly thrive.

Partner up and make a plan.

In order to work together, it is important to sometimes decide a number of things ahead of time. Consider how you are going to plan your cycle. Meaning, does one of you work more and the other go to all of the appointments? It's almost impossible to be all things to each other at all times. Here are some things to discuss and consider:

- Where will you give, take and meet in the middle?

- How will you nurture each other through this?

- What will you do to avoid baby-making burnout?

- How will you handle uncomfortable settings?

- How can you use your unique personalities and strengths to help each other?

- What does the word "helping" mean to each of you?

- When you need help from one another, how will you let each other know?

- How are you going to handle differences in opinion?

- What if one of you is at a stage that the other person is not? How will you handle that?

- How committed are you to following your path?

- How are you going to include others?

- Who will those others be?

- How are you going to handle the financial aspects of your journey?

- At what point will one of you have to return to work if you are currently not working in order for you to achieve your goal?

- How committed are you to following a budget so that you can afford what you are saving for?

- How will you handle purchasing your must haves? Your luxuries?

- What measures do you agree to take if your relationship becomes strained? If your hope fades?

Don't worry if you don't have answers to all of these questions right now. Just start somewhere. Having any sort of a plan will help to keep you moving forward and hoping together.

Give your relationship what it needs to be strong.

When battling infertility issues, relationships can become tired, run down, and sick. Like having a cold, or even the flu, it's about giving your partnership what it needs to be strong. For starters, try respecting each other's style. You are both different. You both respond to things differently. And to top it off, men and women want and need different things.

Even if your relationship right now isn't all sunshine and roses because your baby-making feels more separate than together, and more heavy than happy, it's what's underneath that will get you through your difficulties trying to conceive.

It's important to know what your relationship is made of and how you are each individually constructed. When one of you needs support, what kind of help do you need? Is it the "I just need you to tell me that everything is going to be okay and hug me" kind, or is it the "I need some time to let everything settle in and need some quiet time" kind? What if one of you reaches a breaking point? Will you allow yourselves a temporary breakdown, or will you try to rush in and fix it? Sometimes there is no way to fix it. So what will you do? I had to learn to sometimes hit our hope reset button.

When you've mastered respecting each other's personal styles, start adding in some other relationship reinforcements. What will they be? Will they be late-night cuddlefests? Breakfast in bed? Hope chats? You decide. It's about building yourselves up as a couple. Sometimes this takes time. Start with building slowly. Before you know it you'll be giving each other what you need to be more relationship and baby-making resilient. After all, two are stronger than one. Remind yourselves of this often.

Divide and conquer.

I believe infertility-filled baby-making is best shared. One of you may be more squeamish with needles than the other. One of you may be able to communicate with your doctor better. It all depends on who is comfortable with what. Like a hidden language, it can be a simple understanding between the two of you. Who is the appointment maker and who's the shot giver? Who orders the meds and who walks the dog?

In the beginning it's all about what comes naturally to the both of you. Later you can actually assign roles. It's okay that you may both need each other more now than ever. There is a still a way to find your way together even when you have to be apart. Think of dividing and conquering as way of divvying up tasks and sticking to what you both do best.

I'm someone who feels faint when my blood is taken. I always have to turn my head. My husband on the other hand has no problems with needles. I used to never be able to give myself a shot. Because of my husband's work schedule, though, and because of how far away he worked, my role changed. I became the sole shot giver. I was still not able to do any intramuscular ones, but I was able to do the subcutaneous ones. Our roles sometimes shifted, but we still shared the load.

Think of your significant other the way you would if you were the head chef and they were your sous chef in your kitchen. Your sous chef is really your second in command. Your right-hand person. Your helper. Baby-making, even if it's infertility-filled, doesn't have to be one-hundred-percent hard and one-hundred-percent yours all of the time. It's okay right now if you feel like you are the one doing all of the giving. There will likely come a time when your roles may flip-flop. Like if you have to go on bed rest. It's important not to keep score. It will all even out in the end.

You know the saying "It takes two to tango," well, when it comes to baby-making, if you are so lucky to be riding with a wing-man, it often takes hope times two. Together you are a team, and sometimes one or both of you will have to make sacrifices for the team, even if it's not what you want to necessarily do for yourself. The most important thing to remember is that you are both invest-ing in your future. When you make it, you will both have some incredible hope-filled stories to tell.

Build a retreat.

Retreating to a place that you both can go can help you re-charge and come back stronger after a defeat. One of best things my husband and I ever did to help us cope with our tougher days was to invent something that two four-year-olds might do. We built our very own hideout. It became our fort. Our foxhole. It was our own safe place. The place we would go when we needed to get away from it all, slow the world, and just be. The place where we would go to regain our strength and revive our hope.

Inventing it on a whim, my husband summoned his inner-kid creativity and named it our "Intergalactic Space Defense System" (pronounced igs-dsa). I don't know why we pronounced it that way, we just did. Neither one of us is a huge sci-fi fan, but it just sort of came out. Maybe the movie Star Wars, which we loved as kids, had a little to do with it. After all, one of the prominent features of Star Wars is "the force." I pictured some sort of alternate universe where our force, our hope, surrounded us and bound our seemingly gaping galaxy together. A place where our baby-making abilities were amplified and where we could improve our situation through training with light sabers. We would use it to beat out all of the darkness so that only good things would surround us.

I laugh now when I think about how one fluffy bed, a pile of pillows, one layer of sheets, and a down comforter elicited all of that imagination. But it did. This is the place we needed. We crawled in, hid out, hung out, cried out, dried out, and peeked out when we were ready to take on whatever we were up against. It might sound silly, but this one thing helped me more than I could have ever imagined.

For a long time I rarely took time-out moments for myself, but the day before having to go back for another hysteroscopy, I did. I curled into a ball and hid under the covers. My husband could sense that I was having a difficult time, so he jumped in headfirst and summoned me over to our fort. "I've got your back," he said. "Take cover. All quadrants locked down for safety. Nothing can get us." It took me a few minutes to wipe the tears from my cheeks and to tell myself it was okay to be playful about all that I was afraid of. Once I did, I started feeling the part. "You sure?" I said to him. "I'm sure," he said. "But what if it doesn't work?" "It will," he said. "In time, it will." Then we laughed and cried and stayed there until I was ready to come out.

We later discovered something that we liked to call the "Bat Egg." At the time we were beginning IVF treatment, we lived in a house that had a small circular window above our front door. At night the moon would project an oval shape onto our living room wall above the fireplace. It looked like a giant egg. It lit up the wall and reminded us both of the infamous Bat Signal we knew as kids, the distress signal the Gotham City Police Department used to call for Batman when they needed his assistance. Similar to the large bat emblem that appeared projected on the skies and buildings of Gotham City in times of trouble, our egg also appeared like a giant searchlight.

Even though we didn't have any villains from Gotham City, thank goodness, when our little city of two (three, really, if you count our pup) was in crisis, we liked to think of our Bat Egg as protection from our infertility. It sort of watched over us and looked out for us. It became another hope signal. We were both so sad when we left that house. We always talked about how we wished we could have taken our Bat Egg with us. I hope it's shining on another family in need right now.

Take your hope to go.

Sometimes your hope has to be portable. On one of my more miserable days, I had a doctor's appointment that triggered me unlike any other. I was shaken and upset. I remember getting dressed and thinking to myself that I wished I hadn't told my husband earlier in the day when he asked if I wanted him to go with me, "No, it's okay, I can do this one today by myself, I'll be alright." I obviously wasn't. My husband, I think, heard it in my voice earlier that day. He canceled his lunch plans and decided to surprise me by greeting me in the waiting room. I'll never forget how I just stood there in front of everyone in the office and lit up when I saw him then just melted down and buried my head into his chest. I teared up and used his shirt as tissue. He reminded me of our "ISDS" and said that he'd brought it with him.

That same day, he asked me to lunch to try to cheer me up with my favorite kale salad. I needed all of the super foods I could get, and that sounded good to me. Plus, I suddenly had my superhero next to me, and that alone made me feel stronger. When we were sitting at the restaurant table and before he got up to get a refill of his drink, he carefully laid out all of the silverware on the table and said to me, "Now remember, if anything comes, you have all of these to keep you safe." I realized then that in building our initial fort, we set the stage for building our inner armor. On our hardest days, our hope became our greatest weapon against all that made us afraid.

**Share a teeny bit of laughter together,
even if things aren't funny.**

I ran out of sharps containers (containers designed for the disposal of needles) once so I emptied out a cleaning wipes container, removed the outside wrapping, and asked my husband to draw a picture on it with a permanent marker. You know, just to personalize it for me. To give me something to look at. I figured he'd draw something funny, and I missed laughing with him. He took a marker and drew a picture of our dog doing this funny thing he does that always makes us laugh. After he does his business (trying to be tactful with my description here) he shuffles his feet and digs up big pieces of grass and usually flings it all over the both of us and the sidewalk. You kind of have to be a dog person to get it. It really is amusing to see how intense our dog gets. When other people see him do it, they often cheer him on (so, see, we aren't the only ones who think it's funny).

Anyway, the long and short of it is that my husband drew a picture of him doing that with a grass lawn and some poop on the grass. Once we got over the initial funniness of it all, I found that it still had some light-hearted staying power. Even though I wasn't smiling while giving myself my progesterone in oil shots, I smiled each time I discarded the needle. It helped to ease the pain a little.

Sometimes we found levity in just talking about how things in our infertility-filled world could be different. Improved. Changed. One day while sitting in the waiting area of my doctor's office, I noticed a guy leaning over the counter and whispering to the front desk staff as he dropped off his sperm specimen in the ever-so-familiar paper bag. There's always a slight awkwardness when you see others holding the same bag for apparently the same reason as you. But at the same time there's a slight comfort, too, because you at least don't feel so alone.

This particular gentleman was trying hard not to call attention to himself, but in trying to overcompensate with his whisper, I couldn't help but notice the interaction. I remember thinking, "Wouldn't it be cool if the doctor's office gave their male patients one of those cool metal briefcases to tote the bag in instead?" You know, the kind you see in James Bond films or in the movie Mission Impossible. The ones that make the guy feel strong. Undercover. Unstoppable. A little something so that men could feel a little more empowered toting their specimen in style. It's the adult in them that probably feels like they have to whisper. I wonder what it would do to their ego if it made them feel cool. Would they drop it off with their head held high and say, "Delivery!"

Who knows whether this would make a bit of difference in a man's world or not, but as a woman, I smiled envisioning my man, and any man for that matter, toting their stuff with confidence across the parking lot, into the elevator, and inside of the doctor's office while dropping it off at the front desk.

Whatever you contemplate or imagine together, the point is not really about paper bags or briefcases, per se. It's about occasionally letting your mind wander together. Think of it as a miniature mind vacation that you both take in the moment. It helps keeps your ideas coming and your energy flowing. It keeps you engaged in your daily life and talking about everyday things. Not to mention, it makes the time go faster and helps move you forward.

Above all, love.

Hold each other tight. Give each other a kiss. Hold hands. Cuddle on the couch. Love now. Not later after your baby comes and your family is built, but now. You might feel like you have lost your baby-making spark, but that doesn't mean you have lost your better half or that your better half has lost you.

There are plenty of ways to stay close in your baby-making bunker. Now making love just because might not be at the top of your list right now because it's hard to feel sexy, in the mood, or you just plain can't because of treatment timing issues. Or deeper yet, it might make you feel sad and remind you of all that isn't happening right now between the two of you.

Whatever your current level of intimacy, just be sure to talk. Even though the nature of your infertility means baby-making apart sometimes, your love can and will always keep you together if you let it. And if you are already worrying about what you are going to tell your future child or children when and if they ask you how they were made, because it might not be the romantic story you imagined, just think, you can tell them that the two of you loved each other so much, that before you were even their parents, you planned a treasure map straight to them.

when hope is hard

WHEN IT'S HARD getting pregnant everything becomes hard. It becomes hard to smile. It becomes hard to laugh. It becomes hard to feel hopeful, period. Your hope is up, then down. It's sideways, then backwards. You find yourself moving right along on some days, but other days you're stopped in your baby-making tracks. You worry about allowing yourself to hope too much because sometimes it's tough to believe you're ever going to make it.

When all of the pain inside of your heart keeps you from believing that your world will ever be different, and keeps you from seeing what can still be, it's time to bring your baby-making "bright side" back into focus. Take it from a gal who's been all over her own hope map, there is a way to get back to that place where your hope runs steady and stays strong.

Spark your firefly.

When it's hardest to hope, push everything from your mind and picture a tiny firefly in your hand (or your belly). Fireflies are magical. They are able light their own way.

If you are lucky enough to have seen a firefly buzzing around at dusk, it's like witnessing a tiny miracle right in front of you. Although most male and female fireflies have the ability to fly, some female species are flightless. That's right, they can't fly. This doesn't mean they never find a mate, though. Fireflies are equipped with an amazing feature. They emit light from their lower abdomens and use something called bioluminescence to attract their mate.

There is one type of non-flying adult female that glows brightly and steadily while her flying male counterpart carries a weak and intermittent glow. Yet the two still find each other, and a few days after mating, the female lays her fertilized eggs on or slightly below the surface of the ground. The eggs hatch three to four weeks later. And, yep, you guessed it, baby fireflies are born. This, to me, is truly remarkable. All because of light, Mother Nature finds a way.

Fireflies can remind us that even if some parts of us don't function the same way other people's parts function, we can still overcome our seemingly insurmountable obstacles. Finding, having, and holding onto hope is like holding onto a firefly. We all need hope to light our way so that we can get through to the other side.

Hope is your most important asset if you are serious about getting through all of your TTC troubles. But being and staying hopeful isn't always an easy task. It's sometimes strenuous work. That's why you have to keep a clear picture of your firefly in your mind. When you feel your hope slipping, simply remember her. Spark her glow again. Let her be your hope flashlight when its difficult to see.

Find a hope sign.

If hope is hard, you are probably at a point in your journey where you can't see beyond what is in front of you, around the corner, or what your future holds. As a result, your hope often gets pushed out of sight. When you find yourself battling to keep your hope up, it's time to shoot for your sky before shooting for your stars. This means, go ahead and keep your bigger goal in mind, but remind yourself that big goals are only attained if smaller ones are reached first. So instead of focusing solely on your biggest goal of becoming pregnant, begin focusing on all of the little things that need to happen in order for you to get there. Make sense?

It starts with finding those tiny, sometimes hard-to-see, "hopeful moments" that are woven between all of the baby-making events of your day. It doesn't matter how infertility-filled your daily TTC routine might be. Maybe you look up and notice that the skies are clearing and the sun is shining today, maybe you carry on a hopeful conversation with a good friend, or feel at peace for just a moment. If you don't know what a hope moment looks like or feels like, ask yourself, has there has ever been a time during this process when life looks or feels optimistic again? If the answer is no, keep looking. If the answer is yes, then you've found a hope sign.

Hope signs are all of the little and big things that remind you that all things hopeful are still possible and within reach. All you have to do is locate your first one. Find that one and you'll find another.

Every trooper needs a troop.

Oysters have their bed. Elephants have their herd. Nightingales have their watch. Seals have their pod. Turtles have their bale. And every trying-to-conceive trooper needs her troop. Having a troop is your first and best line of hope defense.

Even though your baby-making abilities, or temporary inabilities, might be as personal and private as they come, baby-makers certainly benefit when they find a baby-making buddy or two. I wasn't very outspoken about my infertility, at first. For my own sake, I needed to keep my private parts a little more private. I didn't realize that keeping things on the quieter side made it harder for me to keep my spirits up. I eventually realized I needed (and wanted) to find a troop.

It's sometimes tempting push people out of your life when you think they won't understand or can't relate, or because you just generally don't feel well and aren't always in good spirits. But just because you don't feel like you used to doesn't mean that cutting off all of the nourishment you got from others before all of this happened to you will make things better. Remember, inviting others to support you can actually be quite helpful to you.

Whatever your troop ends up being, it can be on your terms. You can decide who gets to support your efforts. I am not suggesting that you go and invite the whole world. Maybe it's only a small group of two, three, or four. Inviting a close few into the mix might help with lifting some of the burden. For me, it made a world of difference.

When running your TTC marathon you might gain the most confidence after coming in contact with a crowd of your roaring fans. Or you might run your best after making eye contact with your selected few supporters. Finding another person or couple who has been through what you're going through can be extremely helpful and motivating. Even if they haven't won the battle, maybe they have undergone a treatment that you are considering that you still have questions about. While they might currently already have a newborn or young child and you might not, you may really benefit from hearing how they battled infertility and won or how they made it through something that you are about to go through.

You can also rally a troop online. I'm not saying you need to post your weekly trying-to-conceive updates on Facebook or tweet your daily TTC to-dos on Twitter. Although, if this helps your hope to soar, I say, don't hold back in the slightest. There are several online communities and message boards that are wonderful places to connect with others. Birds of an "infertility" feather definitely flock together, and there is great comfort in finding another person who has experienced or is currently experiencing some of the same things that you are. When you're up for it, reach out. You might be surprised to find there will be others reaching out for you.

Besides having my good friend Erin, I found the heart of my troop through RESOLVE, The National Infertility Association. Joining one of their infertility support groups was one of the single greatest decisions I've ever made. Even during my first-ever meeting, the group and group leader left an imprint on my heart. Her combined strength and resilience was so inspiring. Just having the opportunity to meet and connect with others who get it, and who got me, without having to explain anything was like traveling to an island where everyone spoke my language. I made so many incredible friendships and never felt alone.

This is one of the great ways that RESOLVE impacted my life. They brought people into my life that I would not know otherwise.

If you haven't already checked them out, I urge you to do so. Their website is: http://www.resolve.org/.

RESOLVE is still a huge part of my life. I am still involved and enjoy giving back to the infertility community as a volunteer peer-led support group leader in my local area.

Whether you are more the talkative trying-to-conceive type or not really doesn't matter. The best part about support is that it can be on your own terms. Whether it's confiding in your partner, connecting with a friend who understands, attending a support group, reaching out to your religious leader (if you have one), or talking things over with a therapist, you can include (and not include) whomever you want. Just include someone. Trying to conceive while battling infertility can be a lonely road to travel at times. There's no need to go it alone.

Go Pro.

If you are considering talking things over with a professional infertility counselor or therapist and you don't know where to begin locating one in your area, start with RESOLVE. They have a large number of resources listed under their professional services directory. Besides the peer-led support groups they offer, you may also be able to find a professionally-led support group in your area.

Once you find your core of baby-making buds, no matter how few or many, let them know you hold them in such a special, close regard. Tell them how much their support means to you. And if ever they ask if there is something they can do at that precise moment to help you out, and there is something that would make your life easier, don't be afraid to share it with them. It's entirely okay to do more receiving than giving right now. Trust me, even if you are on the receiving end of support now, you may later find yourself in a giving role able to give back.

Remind yourself why you're doing this.

Even though you're not pregnant yet, doesn't mean that this is the end of the road for you. Every time you feel hope slipping away, try this instead: remind yourself why you are doing this, and that someday your efforts will all be worth it. It can be as simple as saying to your self, "I'm doing this so that someday I will be a parent."

Have a hope phrase.

One way to return to hope is to have a saying that reminds you of it. A phrase like, "Come back." "Return to me." "Here now." Choose a phrase that helps you return to being hopeful. Any time you feel yourself lose your way, go ahead and say it. And, remember to take it to heart.

During hopeless times, negotiate.

When your hope gets pushed away, you are not seeing everything as it is. You are seeing everything in terms of what it feels like in the moment while your hope hides.

If your hope is hiding, talk it out from underneath its cover. If your hope is teetering, talk it down from its ledge. If your hope starts pulling away from you, take its hand and don't let go. Sometimes a hint of hope is all you need to help you start moving again. If you don't give up on your hope, your hope cannot give up on you.

When hope is hardest, one way for you to negotiate with your hope is to visualize it. It's a way of saying, "I see you and I'm not leaving until you come out." In order to do this, think of a time in your life when you were most hopeful. It may be a time before you started trying to have a baby or it might be the time you first began your baby-making journey. What was that time like? What were you like? Visualize that place again. Once you have that image in your mind, try to get back to that place. Visualize your hopeful outcome. Now baby-make from where you are.

When you bring hope to the forefront, you are coming from that place where you are most open. When you proceed as if nothing is wrong, you are able to see everything. Every opportunity. Every happy ever after. I am not saying you should live in denial and pretend that your TTC troubles are a thing of the past. I'm saying that you can benefit when you turn nothing away. Because then, nothing is too painful to keep dreaming of.

Bring hope to your bed rest.

Bed rest is the type of thing you thing that you are often prepared for in your mind, but as it nears and or progresses, you realize it's sometimes harder said than done. Especially, if its not your first time on bed rest. Maybe your thoughts start racing a little. Maybe some of your worries set in. Maybe you used to feel hopeful but are afraid to now.

Don't fret, there are all sorts of ways to inspire your bed rest. While you're lying there, it's important to remind yourself that you are doing everything you can possibly do. You are only in control of so much, and right now you are supposed to be resting. This will give you something to feel good about and help you to think positively.

You can also bring a friend. Have someone wait your wait out with you and help you through it. Whether it's having your dog or cat at your side, if you have one, or having a friend come to watch a movie with you, to bring you a snack or to just sit with you and chat to help take your mind off of things, a little company from a bed rest buddy helps the wait go by faster.

When people ask me how I made it through all of the bed rest during my journey, including all of my two-week-waits and the nine consecutive months of it to get me through to a successful pregnancy, I tell them that while lying there I began thinking about the kind of strength you see in Mother Nature.

I started imagining that I was just like a mama bird whose role it is to sit on my nest for as long as it takes. I called myself that, too. Mama bird. I also told myself that if certain wildlife could somehow adapt and survive despite immense adversity, I could too. So, I envisioned the pregnant polar bears in the Arctic, known for digging out dens on snowy slopes and hibernating there until they deliver their cubs (surprisingly, quite often they deliver twins).

I also pictured the male emperor penguins who endure the freezing cold while incubating and balancing a single fragile egg (their little penguin-to-be) on the tops of their feet to protect it by keeping it off of the ground for nearly three months until it hatches. The thought of hundreds of males huddled together to stay warm made me think of all the other mamas and papas-to-be out there fighting for their little ones. I resigned myself to huddling with those other parents-to-be to stay hopeful even if I didn't know any of them by name.

Be your own best hope.

When hope is hard it's easy to start searching outside of yourself for a hope. I, too, was tempted. The truth is, though, that no one knows how to hope for you better than you do. Even if you are struggling to feel at the top of your hope, trust me, there is no better source of hope than you. When you stick to your own hope, your own hope will stick with you.

One of my friends finds hope by keeping her ultrasound pictures after each IUI by her bed. A second friend finds hope by talking to her mom. And another friend of mine shared with me that at one point the only way she was able to stay hopeful was through unconventional means. The thought of not having a baby one day would eat her up inside, so periodically when she was at a low, she would visit a respected psychic. She tells me it may sound silly, but this gave her hope. All of the sessions revealed to her she would have two kids one day—both boys. Just hearing that it would one day come true allowed her to relax. Then of course she did everything in her power to make it come true. She researched all the ways to make her body healthy. She tried acupuncture and yoga and she drank smelly tea. For her, it all boiled down to doing stuff daily to make it happen. That is what kept her going.

Fast-forward to today. My friend does in fact have two boys now. Both are IVF successes. Coincidence? I guess we will never know for sure. My heart dances for her.

I am not saying you need to visit a psychic to find your hope. In fact, I am suggesting quite the opposite. I see psychics, even so-called legitimate ones, as a very small part of your bigger picture. I only say that because you are your own best hope, and no one, not even a psychic, knows your hope better than you.

If you were to ask me directly if you should go to one, as your new hope friend, first and foremost I would probably advise you to take something of a long, insightful pause before leaping in that particular direction. Infertility has layers. Those layers are often complex and difficult to comprehend. It's tempting to want to find all the answers, but sometimes, just when you think you have an answer, you realize there are no answers. Like in my case, having unexplained infertility.

Even without answers, I don't think you ever need to go outside of yourself to attain your deepest real hope. With that said, though, I would also tell you to follow your heart, and if your heart still points you toward visiting a psychic after your mindful pause, then, as your friend, I of course would support you. I would also tell you to first put your money toward treatment, because that's the real crystal ball for infertility troubles. For most of us, treatment ultimately works.

So what's a fertility-challenged gal to do? The most important thing you will ever do on your journey is to trust your baby-making gut and do what you feel you should do, not what someone else senses or feels you should do.

If you're aching to know more about the whole psychic realm because you're curious, this subject fascinates you, or because you have considered this as an option yourself, I will share my personal experience. This topic occasionally comes up in my support group. If this subject is too out there and not grounded enough in day-to-day baby-making reality, feel free to skip it. No hurt feelings here. I actually thought about leaving this part out, because I don't really see it as a hope essential. I see it more like a hope supplement under the right set of circumstances. Assuming of course that all parties' intentions are clear and you are not looking to put all of your hope in one basket.

As your baby-making buddy, when I set out to write this book, I vowed to myself to be fully open and share my entire experience with you if there is a chance it will help you to have more hope. So here's the story. A dear friend of mine, who lost her beloved husband, paid for me to go to her spiritual medium for a reading. As a widow, her sessions with the medium, gives the life her husband left behind and the one she is left to continue, comfort and meaning.

After the loss of my firstborn twins almost to the finish line (which is something that hopefully you are not going through, or will ever will go through), she wanted to do what she could to make a difference in my search for healing. She wanted to share her experience with me. That the spirits of our loved ones go on.

Before I get into the specifics, it wasn't something I rushed into. My husband expressed his concerns about it with me openly beforehand. He thought that it might mess with my hope more than anything else. I wondered that, too, at the time. Knowing what I know now, I understand where he was coming from. He and I discussed our feelings about it at length, and after my own long mindful pause, I eventually did go. I didn't go because of my infertility. I also didn't go because I wanted to know about babies I didn't have yet. I went because I wanted to know about the babies that I already had, that painfully, were no longer with me.

Visiting the medium actually ended up being really hard for me. I was more nervous than anything else. The entire time I sat there my body was shaking. In some bizarre way, I wanted some sort of sign that my babies were okay. The one thing you learn is that if you do go, it's best to go without any expectations. If you do, you might be disappointed. What you go to talk about might not be what you spend the bulk of your time talking about.

I assumed that the entire session would revolve around my little buns who passed away. It didn't. We talked about other things. Things like health, spirit guides, my husband, relatives and even the fact that my uterus is tilted (which, crazily, it is). It was only at the end of the session that we got to the part that actually brought me there. I remember thinking that it might be my only chance to ask the question that had been plaguing my heart. With my voice trembling I eventually built up the courage to ask the spiritual medium whether or not I would go on to have more children. I was afraid of what she might say. I was also afraid of what she might not say. I wasn't sure if my heart could take any sort of message at all.

After one of the longest, deepest breaths I've ever taken, I was ready to listen, and the spiritual medium answered me. She said that it was as though I had been struck by lightening twice. She said that my husband and I have challenges in front of us, but that we will succeed. She went on to say that she felt confident that he and I were going to fill our two-story home, that I would be pregnant in the spring, and that she wouldn't be surprised if we ended up with twins.

As it turned out, after what seems to be forever, and watching many of our friends go on to have their second child before we could have one living one, my husband and I finally filled our two-story home. After suffering another heartbreaking loss during my second trimester due to a blood clot that formed within me, followed by a failed IVF cycle with my frozen embryos, I got pregnant with the help of IVF again with my husband's sperm and my eggs. Our transfer was at the end of March, and we were pregnant in the spring. And there were two, twin boys. This time fraternal. I couldn't believe that after being sent back to my bunless oven as many times as I had, that my journey finally brought me full circle.

Looking back now, I'm not so sure that going to the spiritual medium made that much of a difference in my actual hope of conceiving. I didn't go there searching for that. It did, however, leave me with a sense of wonder. Life is mysteriously beautiful. It also reinforced what I already knew. My hope for my babies who "passed" combined with my hope for another future pregnancy would have to come from me. I was the one who would have to endure the rigors of treatment, invite the hope into my everyday thoughts and routine, and face any potential risks for future pregnancy complications. Hope is funny that way. It isn't a stand-alone thing. It's connected to every baby-making step we take and every baby-making dream we dream.

All along I think I always knew I came equipped with my own
....-in baby-making magic. After all, even prior to going to the
medium that one time, I kept telling myself I was going to be a
mom. I refused to believe anything other than that. I knew that
meant accepting that I might not become a mom the way I thought
I would.

When all is said and done, if hope is still hard for you at the end
of your day, try to imagine what it would be like if you were helping
your best friend going through the same thing. What would you
say to them? What would you do for them? Now try saying those
same things to yourself. Try doing those things for you. Be the same
kind of hope that you would offer to a dear friend walking in your
same shoes.

hope essentials

REGARDLESS OF YOUR baby-making endeavors, you can always benefit from a short list of "don't leave home without" hope essentials:

Bask in the benefits of being infertility informed.

Knowledge is a requisite for your hope tool kit. Your bunless oven is actually your starting point. Just think, it's most likely one of the reasons that led you to your fertility testing, diagnosis or treatment. Now that you or your partner have been diagnosed, don't let the diagnosis fool you. It contains vital information about you. Imagine, what if there were no such thing as an infertility diagnosis? As much you might hate the infertility word and despise being associated with it, it actually acts like a blueprint, helping to target your problem or problems. It can make all the difference in the success of a cycle and one that involves working aimlessly, alone in the dark.

Armed with your fertility specifics, you may choose (or may have already chosen) to team up with your very own reproductive endocrinologist, whose goal it is to help you make the best possible treatment decisions. Where there are treatment options, there is also hope. It means you actually have a chance to do something about it. The infertility field is always changing and new knowledge and technological advances are constantly becoming available.

When it comes to infertility, I believe it's better to know what you are up against because then something can be done about it. Knowledge is powerful.

It's what we don't know that might actually hurt our chances for success. Your body is unique. It is not like any other. Getting to know your body will keep you from being surprised. As a determined baby-maker, you have already proven to yourself and to others that you are serious about conceiving a child. Now it's time to get serious about making the most intelligent, informed decisions you can possibly make. Informed decisions are capable of leading you to your happily ever after. Sometimes, they can even lead you to your happily ever after faster. Likewise, if you make quick, hasty decisions, you may forget an important step, make a wrong move, or become disoriented and not know which way to go.

Being infertility informed means lots of things. It means doing your own research, learning facts, and finding answers. It means if you don't know what something means, you're not afraid to ask. It means if you think you understand what something means, but have some lingering doubts, you still ask. I found it helpful to write my questions out in advance so that when I sat down with my doctor I could ask away. That way, even if I got tongue-tied or forgot what I wanted to say because I had so much on my mind, I had something to help me remember.

Obtaining accurate and honest information about your infertility plays a role in your trying-to-conceive process. Even if you are presented with bad news, it can be accepted, and new, more realistic goals can be worked into your baby-making. The knowledge you gain can be used to help guide your actions. You often make valuable friendships and pick up valuable tips. Most importantly, you learn how to adapt to your environment, which reduces the fear of the unknown and gives you the best chances of enduring it. Your diagnosis is incredibly important to ensuring that hormone levels are correct and that timing is right to maximize your chances of success.

Strangely, in some ways we should actually give infertility a bit of credit rather than just curse at it. It gets us to take that first step and act. It gets us to move, and in the baby-making world, we've got to keep moving in order to make progress. Infertility tells us what we are up against and leads us to treatments that we can rely upon. When you become infertility informed, you will be surprised how quickly you go from feeling infertility-crazed to baby-maker in charge.

Make peace with your stress.

Perhaps nothing is more stressful than trying for a baby and having it not go well, or go anywhere for that matter. Some of the realities we as bunless oveners have to face are purely stressful right down to the core. I get a kick out of people who think that if we follow their advice and simply "don't stress about it" that we are going to magically become pregnant. It would be great if it were that simple.

While I strongly believe in the mind-body connected powers that be, anyone actually going through infertility knows that it's a medical problem and not a psychological one. There is no way to be a real baby-maker and not stress. That's like telling a mom to never stress. Yeah right. But I do believe you can ease your stress. Not have so much of it. Have less pain, less discomfort, and remove some of the stressors so that you can baby-make with more ease. Your infertility-filled baby-making doesn't have to deplete you. Your infertility can be used to power your steps. All it takes is a stress strategy.

It's true that stress actually makes diamonds. It is a rock's reaction to pressure. Most natural diamonds are formed this way. But too much pressure on your baby-making plate can lead to loss of confidence, difficulty making decisions, anger, forgetfulness, relationship problems, low energy, constant worrying, withdrawing from others, and propensity for mistakes, which can all have a devastating impact on your already tough journey. You cannot maintain a high level of stress indefinitely. It is likely that you would become worn down and a state of exhaustion would set in.

When we're under stress, we have the potential to panic. We might choose to stick with a certain type of treatment that isn't working, or we might prematurely jump into a treatment that we might not be ready for. Stressors, unfortunately, don't always come one at a time. Stressful events often occur for us simultaneously. Stressors add up, and the cumulative effect of them can be very distressing if they all happen too close together.

Everywhere you look these days, the world is going green. In the same way you might already recycle or tote your own reusable grocery bags to the store, and by doing so help to ease the earth's waste problem, there is no reason you can't apply some of the same simple principles to help a stressed sister out—you! By creating your own stress strategy, you can invent ways to reduce your stress.

The first thing you can do is think about anything and everything you can do to make your life easier, and start doing these things one by one. Another thing you can do is to put your stress to work and reuse it for something else, like using it as something to motivate you. Lastly, you can always find ways to recycle your stress and turn it into hope. The goal is not to avoid stress, but to anticipate it and manage it.

That means doing something nice for yourself, just because. Hydrating after you've shed some tears. Offloading just a teeny bit of the stress. You need your body to take you places. Nurture yourself every chance you get. You deserve it.

Learn to say no.

Even when family and friends are accepting of your infertility, you're still bound to have those moments of feeling excluded, when being surrounded by those who conceived with ease, and can't relate to what you're going through.

It's entirely okay to pass on some of your social obligations. You can decline a baby shower invitation. It's okay to pass on attending those get-togethers and gatherings that make you feel sad or going out with other couples with kids. Don't feel like you have to do anything you aren't up to doing. Don't worry, your truest of friends will remain your truest of true pals no matter how many events you might miss. You don't have to take on everything, and it's alright to say no. You're in control of your social calendar. Do what makes you feel most comfortable.

Learn to say yes.

People who survive infertility usually find that at some point they have to learn to say yes to something that they otherwise would have said no to. It's about being open.

The first thought I had about IVF? That's an easy one. It was a flat-out thanks but no thanks. The second time I thought about IVF was an entirely different story. It was during dinner with Erin and her husband, when I met their first IVF miracle. Seeing hope for real changed things for me. There was no label on his little forehead that read "IVF kid." He was just like any other kid. Adorable. Impressionable. Inspiring. A few days after our dinner, I met with our reproductive endocrinologist. Surprisingly, my once firm no became a hopeful, happy yes.

Leave outside influences outside.

When you open up, no matter how hard you try to protect yourself, inevitably it could still happen. Someone will most likely say something that you don't like, or let you down, or you end up feeling more hurt than helped. The thing is that people don't always say the thing that you really want to hear because they don't know what to say. They aren't living your baby-making struggles day to day. You are. So they end up saying the first thing that comes to mind. They might offer up an unsolicited stories about another woman who successfully became pregnant by drinking a certain type of tea, built their family through adoption, or ended up becoming pregnant on their own after years of treatment, which as you know, while well-intended, isn't always the most helpful story to hear in the beginning of your journey.

Ironically, even when we do our best to keep infertility on the downest of down lows, we sometimes still stand the chance of being called out by a naturally occurring secret revealer, time. People can't help themselves. When it comes to baby-making, people ask. That's what they do. Sometimes, even those closest to us fall into the trap of trying to tell us what they think we need.

Here's some of the input I received from people. You might have already heard some of these yourself: "Just relax and it will happen." Little do they know that relaxing hasn't been shown to have an effect on pregnancy rates.

"You can always adopt." Nice. Let's go from zero to a hundred miles per hour in five seconds flat.

"I know someone who did the IUI thing like eight times and it never worked for her." Very encouraging thing to say as I am going through IUI.

"I know someone who was forty-two when she got pregnant for the first time." Um, how about great for her, but what works for one person doesn't always work for someone else.)

"Oh my God, do you have good news for me? Are you pregnant? You would tell me, right? I mean if you were, I would know, right?" Talk about adding some more pressure. I started bawling before she was even done asking.

"You should do yoga." Little do they know that I have been doing yoga for years.

"I read about a couple who drank onion juice and egg whites every day and that worked for them." Hmm, can you say Salmonella and bad breath, how about no thank you.

"I had this dream about a deformed baby." I heard this the day before my pregnancy test. It had nothing to do with me, but I quickly interrupted my friend and said, "Please don't tell me this has to do with a dream about me. I don't want to hear this."

Don't worry even if you think others might be able to flood your focus, influence your decisions, or put a damper on your hope with their comments—you have more control over your baby-making mindset than you know. The trick is to learn to keep your outside influences at bay. The best thing about unhelpful comments is that they can always be erased. You'll find that all the helpful, supportive statements you hear will make up for what the other comments lack.

Speak openly with your infertility insiders.

People generally want to make it better for you by trying to take away the pain. Don't be afraid to let your insiders know that the greatest gift they can give you is to be a listener and a sounding board. Explain to them that instead of erasing the pain, they can help diminish it by their caring. One way to tell your loved ones what you need is to have a simple chat. Begin by acknowledging their comment, thank them for it, and then tell them what you need from them, just like this:

Your friend says:	"You can always adopt you know."
You can always say:	"Thanks for trying to help. I know that's an option. As someone close to me, I am sure you can understand that I have always wanted to be a mom and never thought it would be anything but easy for me to get there. Right now I have to take this process one day at a time and just be where I am. I am not necessarily opposed to adopting, I just want to do everything in my power first before I go that route. What would help me more than anything is if you could be there to just listen and be there as a shoulder for me to cry on right now while I am figuring out my next steps."
Your friend says:	"My friend went through the exact same thing you are going through, and can you believe that after all of

her treatments she got pregnant on her own. If you want I can give you her number so that you can talk with her about what she did."

You can always say: "It's very sweet of you to try to help. Right now I'd like to take a rain check. I am just sticking to the plan my doctor and I have for me. But if in the future I feel the need to reach out to them, then at that time I will come to you for their number."

Your friend says: "I know someone who did that IUI thing you are doing like eight times and it never worked for her. She went onto to IVF and got pregnant that way."

You can always say: "Thank you for trying to be helpful by telling me a success story you know about. The doctors tell me that the process is really very different for everyone, and what works for one person doesn't always necessarily work for another. I am currently on a customized treatment plan specifically for me. We are trying IUI first, which is what our doctor recommends. What I need from you is to just be here with me where I am. It would mean the world to me."

Your friend says: "So-and-so is pregnant. She is wondering if she is going to have a boy or a girl."

You can always say: "Hey, friend, I am sorry, but I can't hear or talk about other's people's pregnancy news right now. It's just too hard for me. I am happy for her, but just sad for me you know."

Another way to let your friends and family know what you need is to write them a letter, text or an email. If you're lost for words, just speak from your heart. The words will come to you. I promise. Don't be afraid to comment that you want children badly, but you've run into some stumbling blocks. You can say that you've been trying to catch up to them with regard to having kids, but so far your efforts have been unsuccessful.

If you're looking to keep it simple, you can say that you thought that you'd have good news to share by now, but you don't, so you just want to let them know where things stand.

You can comment that you believe that you've found the right doctor and right treatment plan, and that you aren't looking for any advice giving really.

You can share with them what you really need from them is their reassuring love, prayers, and support to help you through.

You can mention that rather coming to you for updates, you promise to let them know if something changes.

You can note that their love and support means the world to you and you can thank them for being such a wonderful friend.

You can even say that the fertility meds sometimes cause you to feel tired, have migraines, and because of all of the costs associated with your treatment you don't have much extra money to go out right now. Trust me, sometimes your friends just don't know what you're going through until you tell them.

You can ask to meet up with them for an iced tea or a little walk around the block. You can even ask them to keep their fingers crossed for you.

I received this email from a friend of mine: "It's been forever since we last spoke. Just want to see how you're doing? Any kids yet? None on this end. Just wanted to say hi."

Here's what I wrote back: "As for us and kids, well…been try-ing. Have run into a few roadblocks, so now I'm on the fertility injection track (in my stomach yuk!) We very much want to be parents and hope that we will be blessed as parents someday. We've been getting flooded with overwhelming inquiries about what will come of our efforts. The truth is that right now we just don't know. We're committed to letting everyone know, including you, if anything changes. Thank you for asking how we are, and thank you for caring. We could certainly use your positive thoughts and support, and we are very grateful for your friendship. We hope your quest for kiddos runs smoother than ours. Just remember, just because we are having difficulty doesn't mean that you will. I look forward to someday being able to tell you that we finally made it. Love, Sandi."

Once you know what is helpful to hear, you will be able to guide others close to you to say things that you need to hear. Things like, "I am so sorry," "Is there anything I can do?" "I am here if you need me," "Hugs for your ovaries," "I am holding you in my prayers," "I can't imagine going through what you are."

And if that doesn't work, then you can be your own spokesperson and speak to yourself all the words that hope is made of.

Don't let unexplained infertility stop you.

If you don't know the origin of or specific reason for your infertility, it might feel unsettling, but it doesn't have to stop you. As many of you may know, unexplained infertility literally means infertility with unknown causes. So, yes, this means that through no fault of your own you are going to be less in the know than some of your fellow family builders. But, this is not something to fear.

It's widely known that most infertility cases are treated with medical therapies such as medication or surgery, and many people who face infertility, even the unexplained kind, receive treatment and go on to have a baby of their own. Some even go on to have more than one. Believe it, because it's true.

Even though unexplained infertility makes trying to conceive more difficult and takes much of the success out of your hands, it does not mean that success is beyond your reach. While things might not be running as smoothly as you would like them to right now, you will find that your knowledge can empower you to make decisions, consider solutions, and move forward. I didn't let it stop me. You shouldn't let it stop you either.

Expect the unexpected.

I think most of us would do better with all of this infertility stuff if we could still baby-make in a setting where everything was clear-cut. Wouldn't you know, though, the only guarantee with infertility is that nothing is guaranteed.

Even under the most ideal circumstances, our natural ability to create and sustain life is quite unpredictable. From the outside looking in it can seem pretty straightforward. But it takes a series of intricate events that all happen behind-the-scenes. Hormones have to stimulate. Eggs have to be released. Traveling has to occur down a fallopian tube. Sperm has to swim. Fertilization has to occur. It's no wonder we panic. It can be very stressful operating with limited information with compromised body functions where we have limited control and only so many cycles per year.

Even for the best-prepared baby-makers, unanticipated issues are bound to occur. The key is to expect the unexpected and let things ride out naturally while you deal with what you can control directly. If your baby-making is not playing out the way you expected, it doesn't mean it won't turn out. Trust that you are committed to the process and that you are doing your part. Your most important task is to show up open-minded, ready, and willing. This might mean doing something you never thought you'd do. Or, it might mean skipping a month of treatment if your doctor thinks you can get better results by waiting a month.

During one of my IVF cycles I experienced a severe allergic reaction to one of my stimulation medications. It happened out of nowhere. My face and mouth swelled up, I was covered in hives, and I had to visit the emergency room twice in one day for multiple epinephrine shots and steroid therapy. I looked like a Botox experiment gone wrong, even though I'm not a Botox kind of gal.

But I didn't care about how I looked. I was worried about the big stuff—my safety and more importantly, my treatment cycle.

My cycle was the one thing that had to go on if I wanted to have a baby. What if things were called off? What if the steroids interfered with the other steroids I was supposed to soon take for my upcoming retrieval? What if my hives didn't go away and they refused to put me under anesthesia? In my mind I couldn't afford to miss this cycle. I stuck with what my doctors needed me to do and my condition cleared up. My RE switched me to another type of stimulation medication and my cycle proceeded on just fine.

Tidy your baby-making to dos.

Staying on top of your baby-making to-do list isn't always an easy task. But keeping things simple is the root system of hopeful baby-making. Organizing your TTC tasks into simple to-dos keeps things running as smoothly as possible and keeps you moving forward little by little each day. You might not think you have the patience or the time to tidy your baby-making to-dos. You have enough grunt work. The good news is that it is as simple as deciding what you need to do and doing it—then it's done. You will see. All the little details will line up and bring everything together for you.

Having some kind of organization can help you from going crazy during those times when you feel like you are stuck and going nowhere. You may find that checking things off your list can actually bring some relief. It's proof of progress. Diagnostic tests to undergo? Done. Meds to order? Ordered. Surgery to have? Check. Follow-up appointments to make? Made.

Organizing allows you to juggle multiple tasks with more ease, and it means a little forward progress every day. Keeping it simple prepares you to cope with the rigors of infertility. Organizing at times might seem overwhelming, but you'll soon discover that one decision will lead to the next. If you aren't sure where to begin, start with a list. If you have what seems to be an exhaustive list, don't worry. Pick your most immediate and important tasks and work from there. If you are a skilled baby-maker, you already know the drill. Keep on tending to those beautiful tasks of yours.

Once you have your list, evaluate how much time you will have for appointments and treatments. Also factor in your budget and any foreseeable limitations. These constraints do not have to put a damper on your dreams. Ideally, it is important to recognize them in advance so that you can plan accordingly. If you find that your timeline or plan is in any way unrealistic or overcomplicated, you might have to make some adjustments.

Catch your baby-making breath.

I don't know about you, but it's easy to feel guilty if you stop or pause in your treatment. Remember, sometimes it's okay to take a moment and do nothing so that you can catch your breath. When you're overloaded, no one benefits. Whether it's a physical or mental break, just taking time out in general can be all that you need to give yourself the energy to get through your treatment cycle or energize yourself so that you can move on to the next step.

By clearing your calendar or your mind, you are creating a calming environment. Even if it means giving yourself a break for an hour or two a day, this gives you time to keep the hustle and bustle of it all to a minimum and revive your spirit. It can be helpful to set a time limit on when and how much you talk about your infertility challenges with yourself, your partner, family, friends, and others.

There is nothing wrong with talking about your TTC as much as you need to, but just be sure to allow yourself time in the day, whether it's thirty minutes or several hours, to refresh your body, your spirit, and your mind. Taking scheduled breaks is a positive way to give yourself the time you need to unwind, take a breath, and invite the balance in. Where there is balance, there is hope.

Check in with your hope.

Never take your hope for granted. Just because you think your hope is working for you around-the-clock doesn't mean that it necessarily is. This might seem like an obvious insight at first, but you may be surprised to learn, that with all of the long hours you're putting in trying to conceive, you might not be as hopeful in the present moment as you think you are. Most of us expect our hope to last twenty-four hours a day and during month-long stretches. We assume that hoping our greatest hope at the start of our journey will take us all the way through to our happy ending. It would be great if that were true.

In the early days of my treatment it felt like I was always in a hurry and in "infertility-crazed" mode. I would go to my doctor's appointment, then later drive an hour each way to my husband's work so that he could give me my shot, then I'd come home, get on the Internet reading about infertility stuff, and stay up late thinking about it all. Then I'd repeat the same thing the very next day. Most of the time I felt tired and a bit worn down. I began thinking about the fact that if my body was suffering and feeling kind of cruddy, my hope might be too.

When I first started to regularly check in with my hope, I started to realize that if I felt even a hint of feeling bummed, stressed, or worried about my difficulties trying to have a baby that was a sign for me to shift my thoughts or change something that I was doing. If I didn't initially recognize those feelings or ignored them, those feelings would increase and the less hopeful I felt. I learned that even if I wasn't feeling high stress that day that I still had to listen to my hope. My favorite check-in was to silently say something to myself like, "Hey hope, are you still there?" Once I sensed my hope was still with me and hanging on, I would then say to myself, "I know you are hurting today, but I need you." Then I would often follow up by saying, "You are making me stronger."

It's important to pay attention to what your hope is telling you. Your hope is almost always talking to you. If you're like me and have the tendency to push yourself, checking in is even more important because you won't know your hope is suffering until your cycle is pretty far along. It's amazing how much your hope has to say if you're willing to listen. What is your hope telling you, friend?

Make room for hope naps.

Hit the sack, literally. Being overtired can put a damper on your mood and can cause you to be less likely to commit to a hopeful routine. Whether you rest your head, rest your mind, or rest your body, think of rest like scheduling a doctor's appointment—it is a commitment to giving your body what it needs. In the same way the average baker works twelve-hour shifts, is on their feet most of the day, and works late at night, early in the morning, and on weekends too, you know firsthand that dealing with infertility can easily become all-consuming. The visits to the doctor alone require a lot of time and energy. In addition, just allowing your mind and conversations to run with all of this infertility stuff 24/7 can be exhausting. So instead of a caffeine pick-me up, when you begin sensing that you are becoming restless, worn down, or unfocused, plan to quiet your mind, wind down and take that nap, just because. You deserve it. As a well-rested baby-maker in limbo, you'll be more likely to feel better, focus, and make forward progress.

As someone who hardly slows down, I found hope naps to be challenging at first. I often wondered if a mid-afternoon nap would cause a poor night of sleep. My first IVF protocol included taking Lupron. While on it, I experienced hot flashes and insomnia. Because of this, my sleep pattern got off track. I would lie awake most of the night and rise early, leaving me exhausted during the day due to lack of sleep. I didn't have this problem with my subsequent IVF cycles. I was given Cetrotide. But my Lupron days taught me a valuable lesson: it is okay to rest. When I began to listen to my body and take time for naps, both my body and my hope felt reinvigorated.

Build up your baby-making resilience.

The uphill of infertility is sometimes steep. With great challenges come choices: the choice to stand still, the choice to surrender, or the choice to press on. Find the part of you whose hope isn't clouded. Whose energy goes more to your plan of action than your panic. Whose strength of character includes a mental base layer made of both patience and persistence. Whose determination helps you make it through and out of your tough infertility spots, with your hopes and dreams and self still intact.

Trust me, in the beginning I was more resistant than resilient. Being somewhat of a treatmentphobe, it took a lot of self-encouraging on my part. But I was determined. I knew what I was doing had a purpose. I knew it wasn't just about today's battle. I knew it might also be about tomorrow's. I knew I was meant to be a mom.

In building up the stronger parts of myself I was able to carry the weaker parts of myself. I never saw defeat as an option. You, too, can use your natural gifts to maximize your chances of coming through your infertility to the other side. It feels good to feel your own strength!

The next time you begin to feel like you're drowning because your baby-making tidal waves are crashing down on you and rolling in one after the next, float until your water is calm. Then paddle until you're ready to swim your butt off. Your resilience will save you, I promise.

hoping too soon

IT'S EASY TO get caught in the trap of trying not to hope too soon. Maybe you've just started another treatment cycle after several that have failed and you don't want to somehow jinx this particular one. Or maybe you've received word that you're treatment cycle worked and you're finally pregnant, but you are trying to keep yourself from jumping for joy because you know you aren't so called "out of the woods." Or maybe you've picked out a room in your home as your future baby's nursery, but you keep the door closed because it hurts to plan a nursery when there is no expected due date.

Whatever the case may be it makes perfect sense to think that hoping too soon or too much might ruin your chances of attaining your happy ever after.

There's no such thing as jinxing yourself out of a family because you hoped too soon or too much. The idea that you should stop yourself from "hoping too soon," or "hoping too much," is rooted in whatever fears you may have about your worst-case scenario. It's embedded in your concern that your hopeful outcome might not work out. The anticipation of that outcome hurts you, so it stops you from hoping in your tracks. With this mindset, you go from acknowledging your hope, to denying it.

As much as you might think that hoping early on can hamper your chances of success, you've got it all wrong. Tapping into your hope, and rescuing it from your fears is the same thing as finding your strength. Allowing even the tiniest hints of hope can actually sustain you. During the rigors of treatment, you need that. Hope is what keeps you moving. The next time you sense your mind toying with these notions, have no fear, there are so many things for you to still be hopeful about that you don't have to give up on just because you're not pregnant yet.

I'm not suggesting that if you hope your cycle will be successful that it will be. I'm saying that if you leave room for a hopeful outcome to happen, then it just might happen because you're open to it. And when it comes to those nursery plans of yours, I'm not advising that you should go out, splurge and fully decorate the room you've picked out for your future baby. I'm saying, that instead of completely closing that door because it's too painful to look at, keep the door slightly cracked or place one small hopeful thing in the room or on the closet shelf. Or, when you find yourself dreaming of how your nursery will someday look, save an image to a virtual design board or pin it on Pintrest. Small acts to keep your hope flowing.

It's your dream girl, why not have as much hope as possible?

hope while high-risk

Many things can put your pregnancy at high-risk. Whether you're toting your high-risk pregnancy status because you're carrying multiples, or you're considered to be of advanced maternal age (over the age of 35), or you have a medical condition that existed before your pregnancy, or you've developed a pregnancy complication, or you've had prior poor pregnancy outcomes, you're not alone. There is a whole new era of us mommies-to-be out there whose pregnancies need additional and specialized attention. I say the word us, because I was there.

As if just being high-risk from the start isn't hard enough, carrying all of the added risks can be quite overwhelming. I've felt many of the same fears you might be feeling. While pregnant with Brecken and Caden, I had placenta previa, an incompetent cervix, and carried the MTHFR C677T gene mutation. I underwent a cervical cerclage, took L-methylfolate, special B6 and B12 vitamins and baby aspirin, and gave myself daily Lovenox shots (that later switched to Heparin injections as my due date neared). I also had to limit my activities and stay put for nine straight months of bed rest. I wasn't able to go for walks, do prenatal yoga, or go on a babymoon, that ever so popular final trip that expecting mamas and dadas sometimes take before their newborn arrives. And while I missed out on a normal pregnancy, I knew the importance of following my doctor's instructions because every week was a step forward for my babies.

Don't be fooled by the phrase.

Having your pregnancy being called "high-risk" may sound scary. After all, your pregnancy is considered to be complicated. But, just because you are at high risk doesn't mean that you or your baby will have problems. It's just a way to make sure your doctor will be watching you closely so that they can find any problems early, if any do appear. If any do, you will be able to get the care you need when you need it.

Accept that you're special.

While high-risk, it's important to remind yourself that your pregnancy is getting special attention. Instead of seeing it as a bad thing, try to think of your pregnancy as a VIP. A VIP is a Very Important Pregnancy. And as a member of the VIP Club, you can expect to be treated like one.

This means you will be monitored more closely, you will have more visits to the doctor, and you will have more ultrasound tests to make sure that your pregnancy is going well. You may be cared for by your regular OB and occasionally have consults with a High-Risk OB, or you may be cared for by a perinatologist with specialized training in maternal fetal medicine and high-risk pregnancy complications. In short, you can expect a level of specialized care that "regular" pregnancies simply can't get access to. Pretty sweet, right?

Ask, ask and ask away.

You're bound to have questions about your high-risk condition. If you do, ask them. Even if you can't think of any questions, ask your doctor to repeat what they just said so that you can have a conversation together about your next steps. Don't be afraid to start asking. You can never ask too much.

Because I wanted to know all of the possibilities, the consequences and things to expect, I'd often bring my questions scribbled on a notepad so that I would remember to ask them during my visit. Sometimes a question that might seem unimportant to you might help your doctor help you better.

Have a high-risk buddy.

As a high-risk mom-to-be, at some point in your pregnancy, you might need or want a shoulder to lean on. Whether it's having your partner at your side during your appointments, your pet resting beside you when you sleep, a close friend or family member that comes over once a week, or another high-risk mama. There are all sorts of people around you who I am sure would be there for you in a heartbeat. You just have to ask.

When one of my friends was pregnant with her twins and began having some "panicky moments" toward the end of her pregnancy, I reached out to her. Being that I had survived my own high-risk ordeal, I had a sense that she might need a sounding board. It wasn't long and we began texting back and forth daily. I'm happy to say she went on to safely deliver her twins on time.

If you would like some support and don't know anyone else who is or has been high-risk, you can always find support through an online community or a message board or by contacting Sidelines, a non-profit organization that offers international support to high-risk expecting mothers and their families.

hope after loss

MY ONGOING WISH and my prayer is that no one will ever suffer any sort of pregnancy loss or infant loss, but should you ever need this chapter, it's always here for you. May my personal story wrap and console your grieving heart, provide you compassionate company from someone who "gets it" and "gets you," and above all offer you a true glimpse of hope after loss.

Heartbreakingly, some of us lose some of our baby-making battles before we win any. We become pregnant with the help of fertility treatment but later go on to experience a loss or losses. Our little one or ones go on a step ahead of where we are. Time stands still. All hope seems lost, and life as it used to be is never the same.

Some of us have only our first ultrasound pictures and nursery dreams to take with us. Others of us have our mommy memories filled with first heartbeats, first kicks and first hiccups, followed by the unthinkable. We suffer a loss only weeks or even days before we should have delivered a healthy newborn or newborns. We have to go on with delivering our baby or babies as though nothing ever happened. When it's all over, instead of getting to hear that first cry, we get a few tiny moments to hold our little one or ones with eyes closed to say goodbye when we never even got to say hello in person. All we take home with us are empty hospital baby blankets, a couple of photographs and the little knit beanies that our babies wore. Some of us also leave with belly scars and breast milk already "in".

No matter what type of loss you have faced, we all share a similar dream. The dream that although there will never be a replacement for our first little bun or buns, we want to try again for children. We want to resume treatment, but with all of the pain in our hearts, we have no idea how we are going to survive our possible attempts to come. We knew our hope before, but we don't know how to hope after losing all that we once had.

For some of us it truly is a longer road. My husband and I had every reason in the beginning to believe that we ultimately became part of the group of lucky ones on the infertility treatment block. We finally became pregnant with our first round of IVF. As I mentioned earlier, prior to that, we had endured four failed cycles on Clomid, and four failed IUIs after undergoing laparoscopic surgery to remove a rare uterine mass from my uterus and slight endometriosis on my ovaries. So, you can imagine that once one of our day-three embryos took and implanted and later split, we soaked up every minute of our newfound miracle times two, our identical twins. We could hardly believe it. We thought the hardest part was over and our hearts danced and celebrated.

Soon enough it started to feel real, as my pregnancy hormones were in full effect. Multiplied by two, I felt dreadfully but gratefully nauseous. Forget morning sickness—I had all day sickness. But nothing could keep me from smiling as I was finally toting my buns-to-be. Early in our pregnancy I was diagnosed with placenta previa, a pregnancy complication in which my placenta was covering my cervix. Our doctor assured us that most of the time this complication resolves itself. I was scared, but it did. But just as life was finally coming together for us and we were well on our pregnant way, at twenty weeks (eighteen weeks until our C-section), I was admitted to the hospital for preterm labor, an incompetent cervix, umbilical cord prolapse, and possible preterm premature rupture of membranes of one of our twin son's amniotic sacs. Just like that, things went from feeling hopeful to feeling helpless again.

I was placed in what is known as the Trendelenburg position in my hospital bed. Basically you are lying flat with your feet higher than your head. The idea is that gravity will help keep the babies stay put. I soon underwent an emergency cerclage (a cervical stitch that is placed in and around the cervix to help hold the babies in longer) because my cervix was slightly open. This is known as "cervical incompetence." In addition, I was treated for umbilical cord prolapse, an emergency with the umbilical cord that imminently endangers the life of fetuses. My umbilical cord was beginning to come out, so it had to be pushed back in to remove the pressure from the cord. The doctors also suspected preterm rupture of one of my amniotic sacs since I experienced the feeling of fluid leaking, a potential sign of water breaking.

After my cerclage was performed things seemed to be serious but somewhat stabilized. I was determined to make it to the most important milestone that there is when it comes to having a baby: carrying to at least twenty-four weeks gestation. This is the earliest possible date that our doctors would deliver our twins to give them the best fighting chance. When carrying twins, you are considered full-term at thirty-eight weeks instead of the standard forty weeks for a singleton.

This so-called safe date became my sole focus. I pictured us making it to this date. I received shots of terbutaline almost every hour on the hour to try to help stop my contractions. If you have ever been prescribed terbutaline, then you know how much it causes your heart to race rapidly and what a scary feeling it is to feel like your heart is jumping out of your body. Terbutaline is no longer given beyond 48–72 hours to treat preterm labor and now carries with it warnings because of the potential for serious maternal heart problems and death. Geez, I was on it for weeks.

From my hospital bed I ran on little sleep, but it didn't matter, because I was now in fight-for-life mode, and I wasn't about to let my babies go anywhere. I made it sixteen days lying there without getting up a single time, trying with everything that I am to try to change fate from my hospital bed. When I was at the twenty-two-week mark, I was convinced we'd make it, because after all, we'd made it this far and I only had ten more days to go.

On my sixteenth day of hospital bed rest, though, things took a turn for the worse. Our doctors began preparing us to lose one of our twin sons. It was our Ryan, whose sac is the one they suspect ruptured. This allowed an infection to come in. The ultrasound showed the presence of ascites, an accumulation of fluid around his heart. My little boy was suddenly in trouble and there was nothing that I could do to help him or save him. We were told our one twin who's sac ruptured wouldn't survive the ten day wait, but our other son was in perfect health and holding on.

Facing our son's impending death was unimaginable to me. I couldn't even wrap my head or heart around the idea. After all, I was still carrying him. I couldn't even think of letting him go. I was heartbroken and horrified. I would have to go on fighting for our other son's life all the while with Ryan passing away. The doctors assured us that we could continue on fighting our preterm labor and continue with our pregnancy with his brother Brayden, since he was in a separate sac. They explained to us that such a thing was possible, though not without risks.

I closed my eyes momentarily because they hurt and were beginning to swell from crying so hard. I pictured our two cribs and our double jogging stroller and I couldn't help but continue sobbing. The thought of not filling them both was hard to believe. I was absolutely devastated. I knew I had to reel in my tears somehow and pull myself together to keep fighting for Brayden. I was worried that crying so hard was going to cause more contractions. I kept telling myself that I would get to cry my cry later.

I didn't know how I was going to do it, but I knew I had to temporarily bury my tears to give Brayden a fighting chance. It felt like part of me was being buried alive. I was choking on my breath and my tears all at once. I had no words. Everything hurt. I wasn't going to get to say hello or goodbye to Ryan the way I wanted to. My two dreams come true were suddenly going to become only one. With tears falling down on my belly, all I could say to them was "I'm trying so hard."

Even though Brayden and I weren't out of the woods yet, his strong heartbeat was the one thing that gave me the strength to go on and keep fighting even though I was going to lose my other little boy. It was almost impossible to rest or sleep that night. I had been trying to fight back my tears for hours and I wanted to stay up all night with my little guys. Exhausted, I finally drifted off to sleep.

In the morning our doctor performed another ultrasound. In an instant we went from being the luckiest parents to the unluckiest parents on the labor and delivery floor of the hospital. I could tell from our doctor's face that something had gone terribly wrong. I think all that he said were the words "I am sorry." That is all that I heard. At that moment, I felt all of my strength leave me. It is a feeling that will never leave me. My grief at this point was unbearable. All that I had loved and fought so hard for had been taken from me. I was totally devastated and unprepared for the news that sometime in the night both of our boys had passed away together. Even though our sons were in separate placentas, because of the whole unique nature of twin pregnancies, twins sometimes share blood vessels throughout the uterus. That's what happened to us. Because our one little guy was having difficulty with a ruptured sac, we ended up losing both.

My pain and suffering was brand new again. Just as I was trying to wrap my aching heart around how I could live without my one, I suddenly was thrust into having to go on living without my two. My baby boys that I thought in my heart would be delivered to term would not be. The tiny pitter-patters of their twin heartbeats I was so used to hearing on the fetal monitoring machine I would never hear again. It was the saddest day of my life.

I couldn't turn my head off. I kept thinking of all of the what ifs. What if I had gotten to the hospital sooner? What if I had demanded a cerclage instead of just politely inquiring about it the way I did early in my pregnancy? What if I hadn't climbed the stairs? What if they had measured my cervix sooner? From that moment on, I was no longer me. My hopes and my dreams that were right in front of me all became one great big what if. All the hope I had been carrying suddenly ceased to be. Just like that. It was over. We had our C-section that day, but instead of it being the joyous moment I had always dreamed it would be, it was the worst, most awful, most heart-wrenching day of my life.

All of the moments following my surgery felt like watching a movie of someone else's life. I didn't recognize myself, my life, and I didn't understand. All that had happened was incomprehensible. The hospital's social worker was scheduled to come by to discuss arrangements. The thought of that was inconceivable to me. I told my husband I didn't want to meet with her and that I wanted us to make the arrangements on our own. Due to even more complications, I couldn't even fully grieve the loss of my boys until I physically recovered. In addition to a C-section infection and maternal anemia, I became septic.

We weren't able to have a funeral because I was in bad medical shape and had to remain in the hospital for another couple of weeks. For several days we remained on the labor and delivery floor listening to everyone else's babies being born. Everyone else's dreams being realized. Everyone else's but ours. I was eventually moved to another floor. Another depressing floor. I was with all of the critically ill patients. I wanted out of there, but my body and doctor wouldn't let me until my infections were under control.

My husband had to go to the mortuary without me. No mom, and I mean no mom, should ever have to miss their child or children's funeral arrangements, but I had to. It was so hurtful and life had already been so unfair. My mom, dad, and in-laws came to see us during this time. They were the only ones I wanted there. They were the only ones who saw the boys bundled before they had to go. I didn't know how to face the rest of the world, let alone myself. Here we were, family, coming together for all of the wrong reasons.

My husband brought our sons' ashes back to me in a silver heart-shaped locket that both of our moms picked out for us when they were visiting. I couldn't believe that was all I was going to leave with. How did I go from being a blessed mommy to a sickly skeleton? My belly scar, our hospital bracelets, two baby beanies, and some photographs were the only signs I had left that my boys had ever lived and been with me. I cried the entire night that first night in the hospital and all the days and nights after. I had nightmare after nightmare, and I never thought I would feel peace again. I knew I was never going to be the same. We had finally become parents, and our twisted fate took all of it away.

Our pastor, who was a personal friend, and had really only been our pastor that one time, also came to see us. My husband and I are both spiritual people and have faith in things much larger than ourselves, but we are not deeply religious by any means. At that moment, nothing, not even faith, seemed to matter to me. I just wanted to talk to someone who was closer to God than I was at that moment. I was keeping my distance on purpose. I was angry. I didn't know why he chose me, if there is such a thing as that.

I remember telling our pastor that I must have been a horrible person to have this happen. He reassured me that terrible things sometimes happen to even the kindest people. He sat with me and held my hand. I pleaded with him to help take the pain away. I pleaded with him to help me understand.

I bared my soul and told him the story about the nightmare I had just had the night before. Telling it, I cried to the point where I was almost inconsolable. I had dreamed that I was lying on an operating table and my husband was draped over me sobbing. There were ladybugs all around me. On the table, on me, they were everywhere. I remember the doctors wanting to call someone on the phone, but I don't remember who they were trying to call. I think they were discussing isolating me or quarantining me until they could figure out the ladybug situation. After that, I don't remember much. I just remember that the thought of ladybugs, which I used to love as a little girl, suddenly filled me with despair.

It's strange how the brain works. It has the ability to remember and pair two unrelated things that share a common element and make a once-happy memory a new sad one. My pastor shared another point of view with me. He suggested that maybe the ladybugs were like angels. Seeing to it that my boys were safe. I wasn't ready for that kind of acceptance. Later that acceptance grew.

I had two more encounters with ladybugs that summer. The first was when my husband and I traveled to heal and spend time with family. We leisurely hiked up Green Mountain in Boulder, Colorado. When were almost to the top, a young boy followed by his father came running down the mountain screaming. He was excited. He told us there were ladybugs at the top. Hundreds of them. The news instantly hit me like a ton of bricks. I started to cry. How could it be that on the very same day and trip, I was trying to get away I couldn't? I desperately needed to escape, but it was as if the Universe wouldn't let me.

I didn't know it at the time, but in late summer, the mountains are the destination for the annual ladybug migration. According to naturalists, this is an annual event, although the year I was up there, at its peak there were more ladybugs than experts had seen in a long time. If I had known this, I wouldn't have hiked that day.

My mom was the only one who instantly made the connection between me and the ladybugs. Her eye contact said it all. She must have remembered me telling her the story about my dream in the hospital. She had also been there during my last ladybug freak-out when the hospital staff brought me a plastic bag to put my clothes in that had red ladybugs printed on it. Knowing that the ladybugs are a painful sight for me, she said, "I am so sorry sweetie. I had no idea." I told her it wasn't her fault. "You don't have to go up there if you don't want to. I will stay with you," she said. I told her, "No, I'll go." Life was flooding me with ladybugs at every turn and I was growing tired of being mad at something I used to love.

When I got to the top of the mountain, I didn't stay long. In fact, I think I counted to three, and then I was outta there. My family was taking pictures, like all the other normal people up there, all enjoying the colorful event in awe. Ladybugs covered every rock, every tree, and all of the ground. They were everywhere. I could feel the tears streaming down my cheeks, and I was trying to be mindful of my steps. I didn't want to step on any ladybugs and I didn't want any to land on me. I was doing everything I could to guard my body and my grieving heart. It was so unnatural for me to avoid the one thing I used to associate with luck.

Then it began to rain. I turned and started to run down the mountain as fast as I could. I made it almost the entire way down running. My husband I think eventually caught up with me. I had his dog tags with me. The ones I had engraved for him for Father's Day. Out of breath, I kneeled down, held them close to some wildflowers, snapped a photo with my phone. I was getting drenched but I didn't care. The raindrops were holding me and I let them.

Not too long after we returned home, I had my second ladybug encounter while out on a walk with our dog Jake. I stopped to look at a cluster of kangaroo paws, the same kind of flower I planted to honor our firstborn sons. It was then that I noticed that they were next to a tree with bright purple blooms all over it. On the stems of that tree were ladybugs. Again, they were everywhere. It was strange because they were only on that one tree and nowhere else. I made a daily ritual of walking that same path so that I could return the tree until one day the ladybugs were no longer there.

Since then my relationship with ladybugs has become much more powerful, softer, and reflective. Maybe if there is such a thing as a sign, maybe I got the initial ladybug sign wrong. Maybe it wasn't meant to devastate me. Maybe it was meant to tell me that things weren't as they seemed. That maybe death isn't death. Maybe with life comes a veil. Maybe in some way with loss comes some kind of hope, says the girl who couldn't see anything hopeful when I returned home from the hospital.

"I don't know how to do this," I remember saying while sobbing to my husband over and over in the car as we drove up our street and arrived back at home. The same place where we last lived happily together. The place where our nursery waited for our boys' arrival. The place where all of our neighbors last saw me toting our twosome. I didn't want to get out of the car, but I didn't want to stay there either. When I got inside, everywhere I looked reminded me of them.

The first thing I did was crawl under our covers on our bed. It was all I was physically and mentally capable of doing. I wanted to just hide, if that's what you would call it. I didn't care if anyone was looking for me. At that moment I could not be found. I think I even put the blankets over my head, and I never do that. But then again I wasn't me anymore so I am not surprised that I did something out of the ordinary. Habits no longer mattered. I didn't want to do anything. I didn't want to talk to anyone. Nada. I just wanted to be in a ball with my blankets. The place I had last been pregnant. The place I had last been their mom. That's the only place I could collapse in a world that just collapsed on me.

When I was in the hospital on bed rest with our firstborn twins, I would sing Hawaiian songs to them every day, sometimes all day. I don't know why really. I don't listen to Hawaiian music at home, and the last time I heard Hawaiian music was at my wedding. There was something about Hawaiian music, though, that helped me be as calm as I could be given the circumstances. My heart gravitated to it. Maybe it was prompted by the fact that my husband brought me a photograph of our wedding day and put it next to me on my hospital room wall. I just remember lying there wishing I could hear the same ukulele that played IZ's "Somewhere Over the Rainbow" during our wedding ceremony. Being a musical soul prior to our boys passing, I could never picture life without music. But being a grieving mother trumped all of that. With our boys gone, I felt that I would never hear music the same way again. My life seemed noteless.

Strangely, within a couple of hours in my bedroom hideaway, I started humming a tune I had never heard before. It kind of landed on me the way a butterfly would, and it just kind of sat with me and kept me company. I longed to be alone, but at the same time I was okay with it being there. I eventually popped my head out from underneath the blanket I was curled up in when my husband came to check on me. I either gestured for or asked my husband to bring me a notepad and pen. He did, and not too long after that, I wrote our boys a lullaby out of words that seemed to come out of nowhere. To write it was as natural to me as breathing. All I can say is that for some reason the tune felt purposeful.

Rather than trying to make sense of the song, I just went with it. After all, nothing made any sense to me. My boys weren't with me. I was at my hope tipping point, and I had no words. I folded the piece of paper with so-called lyrics and placed it underneath my pillow and kept it there.

A few days later my friend Donna came to the house. She was the first friend to come visit me in my bedroom hideout. I couldn't say much, but I told her about the song. When it came time for her to go, she hugged me goodbye, I cried, and she urged me to find a translation dictionary. I managed to locate one online. I plugged each word in to the translation text box and for all but one word that I sang I found a corresponding word in Polynesian. Also known as Hawaiian. I wrote them all down. Not sure of the correct spelling, of course.

What came next surprised me. Within the translated words were themes that bore a striking resemblance to my loss. There were parts about one who tries to understand. Parts about being surrounded by emotion. Parts about a period of pregnancy ending. Parts about closed lips that make no sound. Parts about searching for calm and relief of pain, and parts about a sharp pain in the stomach scarring over. As a grieving forever mommy who could say nothing because it felt like all of my words had left me, I was reading words that I deeply felt but could not and did not know how to let out.

I realize it may be wishful thinking, but I like to think of it as the lullaby that came to me to let me know that my boys are somehow somewhere okay. For me, it remains something that requires no real proof of course. It was a special little song that came to me in its own special way at a time when I was not able to communicate with words. It was just what my aching heart needed to hear at that very moment. It opened my heart to hope again. To this day I have never hummed another song or written another one like it.

A few years have passed, and my husband just recently gave me a guitar as a gift. He knows the musical side of me has been longing to bring more music into our lives. Maybe someday the song will return. I kind of don't think so, though.

Since then, my sons Brecken and Caden have been born and new songs have found me, but that folded piece of paper remains one of the most treasured things that I own. Even though, to a great extent, I am a see-it-to-believe-it kind of gal, I just have to trust that some things in life, like a lullaby that effortlessly just drifts in, that can cause you to feel hope when you have none, need no further explanation. Maybe hope travels farther than we know. I like to think so.

The hopeful tune of my boys' song unfortunately faded into the background as I spent the next several months in and out of bed, having a nurse come to our home to pack and unpack my C-section incision so that it could heal from the inside out. It was a painful process and I could feel that it would be a long while before I felt hope again.

I was on antibiotics to help wipe out the blood infection that I developed, and they made me feel sick. I wanted off of the meds. I had had enough meds, but I had to keep taking them if I wanted to get better. The part of me where my sons had been that I didn't need anyone touching or seeing, let alone messing with, was constantly being reopened. I kept reliving what happened and reliving trying to save them. I stayed in our bedroom, in pain. I was unable to do much of anything. Our friends were as supportive as they could be, but nothing helped. I needed to heal. I needed time.

I had to learn to stop searching for answers that could not be found. We had such big plans and dreams for us and for our boys, and we were almost to the finish line! We did all the right things, made it to all of our high-risk perinatologist visits, and hit every milestone. But complications are just that. They are complicated. No one really knows why some things happen to some people and why others safely dodge the same sequence of events.

We never expected that Twin-to-Twin Transfusion Syndrome (TTTS), a disease that affects many families who are pregnant with multiples, would arise out of the infection that was introduced all because of my ruptured sac. Even though our other son's sac was still intact and he was doing well, and both of our boys were genetically fine, it still took their lives just ten days before their safe date. During our C-section it was revealed that my two placentas were fused, so when our one son starting having trouble due to the infection, because of one or more behind-the-scenes shared blood vessels, as brothers, they went together.

The hardest part about their death was figuring out how to go on without them. We had to live in the same house. See the same neighbors who last saw us with a big pregnant belly. Sleep in the same bed where my amniotic sac was leaking. Do all the same things without our dreams come true by our side. Silence was the only thing I was capable of.

Eventually I built up to a few sentences a day. That time seems like a blur. My mother-in-law came to care for me since my husband had to leave town for training. I was so glad she was there, but at the same time I could not escape the ghost of the daughter-in-law I once was, the expectant one. I had planned to give her grandchildren to hold, to love, and to watch grow. The way I know she wanted to hold them. Love them. Be part of their lives. The reminder was painful for both of us. We just hung out together and cried together, and then she left. It was the best and worst visit we ever had.

People meant well, but one by one they would all fall into the same trap of telling me that there must have been some greater reason, because that's just the thing that people say who have never suffered a loss. I think people in general just don't know how to handle tragedy, especially when it involves babies. I can't really fault them for saying something so removed and stupid.

To this day, with every inch of me, I still personally disagree with the notion that the loss of a child is part of some grand plan. This explanation of things is overused and it's popular, and it seems to be the only thing that pops into people's minds at that uncomfortable moment of silence. While that might hold true for some situations and for some people, when the doctors explained to me that there was something like a 1 in 50 million chance of the exact events that followed my rupture of membranes occurring, you can't tell me that I am the 1 in 50 million for a planned reason. I love you guys, but you're clueless. If there was such a "grand plan" set out for me, then why this on top of everything else? On top of this I was in bad medical shape. In a way, I am glad that you are clueless because that means you don't know the kind of pain I know. I wouldn't wish that on you even if it meant you could comfort me better.

A couple of weeks after losing my firstborn sons, our friend's three-year-old daughter came to visit me while I was still healing from my infection. She greeted me sweetly and hovered over my belly as if she were a belly fairy. She said to me almost whispering, "Where are your babies?"

While choking on my tears that I could feel building up, and after trying to swallow with the huge lump in my throat, I summoned up all the strength I had to answer her and tell her that our babies were no longer here and no longer with me. Of course, like all three-year-olds do she followed her question with a series of whys. Why aren't they here, she asked? Why can't I see them? I listened as her mom explained to her that my babies weren't ready to come into this world. Why aren't they ready, she asked? Little did she know, I had the very same question.

When I was ready to form words, I told her that hopefully someday I would be so blessed to tell our future baby or babies of their two amazing brothers who fought until they couldn't fight any more. I told her they did what brothers do—they stuck together. One got sick so the other left to care for him. In my dreams they are always together.

I spent a lot of time wishing over and over that there was some way that I could go back in time, get a cerclage, do everything right, and help save our boys. I soon began to realize that no amount of tracing my steps could bring them back to us. Instead, I would have to find a way to go on while still honoring them. Our doctors asked us to wait six months before undergoing another cycle of IVF due to the C-section and the infection my uterus needed to heal from, so we did.

Having a natural concern for the health of any babies we may be so blessed to conceive in the future, we followed their advice. We were encouraged by our perinatologist that it was highly unlikely that we would again confront TTTS and we left our final post-partum appointment with him knowing that I would require a cerclage around fourteen weeks should I get pregnant again. We were told things might go a lot better for us if we were able to get pregnant with just one baby next time. Like we had any control over that!

Losing my two buns at once after holding them in my tummy for six months is the saddest story I've ever had to live and tell. You can imagine that it took me some time before feeling hopeful again. I didn't have the slightest clue how to bounce back into baby-making with hopeful feet first.

We finally set out to give IVF another try. Our treatment protocol was slightly different and called for administering fewer injections, which gave us a little bit of shot reprieve. During bed rest we again found ourselves battling a bundle of nerves, fear, and excitement. The two-week-wait felt like an eternity, again.

Our efforts were successful as we learned that this time we had achieved a pregnancy of one. Things seemed to go really well at first, however, two days before my eleven-week mark I began to bleed. My doctor called it a threatened miscarriage and instructed me over the phone to lie down and to not move.

I was unable to swallow those words, and I was unable to fathom something again going wrong. The very next day I was diagnosed with a subchorionic hematoma (SCH), the pooling of blood be-tween the membrane surrounding the embryo and the uterine wall. Basically it was a blood clot that had formed within me. The doctor informed us that it was something that they frequently saw in IVF pregnancies and that the hematoma would either resolve itself or get bigger, bringing with it an increased risk that I might miscarry even if our baby was genetically fine.

On bed rest I went, only this time it was at home. Here I was counting down again, only this time I was counting down to my upcoming scheduled cerclage, which was scheduled for fourteen weeks, assuming things cleared up. We built a bed on our downstairs floor made of sofa cushions and a top mattress. For twenty days I rested, and with each passing day my SCH appeared to be resolving itself.

When we went in for our next weekly appointment, we were actually expecting our doctor to tell us that things were getting better, but the look on his face was a look that we had seen before. One that told us everything. The look was followed with the words that there was no longer a heartbeat. He explained to us that because we we'd reached this stage of pregnancy I would have to undergo a dilation and evacuation (D&E), a procedure used to dilate the cervix and surgically remove the contents of the uterus. We both sobbed as they let us have the room alone for a while. How could we be here again? Losing again for the third time in a row.

Throughout my three losses (my first twin pregnancy and my singleton pregnancy) I had to learn how to hold myself up and how to live and build my life again without my three most beautiful blessings at my side, carrying them only in my heart. While there is no way to bring my first three buns back, I did find my way to hope again. It took two more IVFs, a cerclage, and nine months of bed rest, four months of which were spent in the hospital.

When we learned we were having twin boys again, at first I couldn't believe what I was hearing or seeing (through my tears) on the ultrasound. My life changed forever (again) that day. It was beyond special for me. It was the first time since the loss of my firstborn twin sons that I felt whole again. I couldn't believe that after being sent back to my bunless oven as many times as I had, that my journey finally brought me full circle. I was speechless. I was so happy to be given another chance. It was extremely difficult to keep all of my worries about my previous pregnancy complications at bay. My fears instantly flooded me.

What got me through? Once I caught my breath, I looked down at my belly and said to my little guys, "We're gonna make it." I knew that strength only came from one place. It was from the strength of my lost little ones' three hearts combined with the hope I was now carrying for their brothers. This strength carried me through nine months of bed rest. I went straight from being on strict bed rest at home to spending the last four months of my pregnancy on strict bed rest in the hospital.

I finally ended up breaking down when I reached full-term and was only a couple of hours away from my scheduled C-section. I was a complete nervous wreck the day of my scheduled delivery. That's when it hit me that it was all happening for real. My wonderful perinatologist was kind enough to have the nurses hook me up to the tocodynamometer (pronounced "toco" for short) just to give me some peace of mind until the surgery. I just focused on their two heartbeats, my own, their occasional hiccups and nothing else.

Every minute until my scheduled C-section felt like an eternity. I begged my perinatologist to pinch me the day it was actually happening for real. Afterward, when it felt too good to be true, he pinched me. I bawled and remember thinking that I hope he gets to pinch every one of his patients like that someday.

In sharing all of this with you, my hope is that you find your way back to the hope you once carried, still carry, and all the future hope you will carry again. Here are some things that I learned along the way:

You're not alone.

There aren't enough words in the English vocabulary to describe what it feels to finally have your baby bump only to suddenly to lose everything you worked so hard for and be sent right back to where you started. You are not alone in fearing that you might have lost the only baby you might ever have, or in questioning yourself if you could have done more to prevent it, or in asking yourself "Why?" over and over again.

The movie stars will have you believe that it is easy to conceive a child or children at any age, and you almost never hear of any of them experiencing a loss. Friends or family members might even have you believing that conceiving a child is a piece of cake, because it might have seemed that way to you. But, behind many people's baby-making scenes lies loss. I was surprised to learn that several of our acquaintances had also experienced a loss. I never knew it because they never talked about it. But then again, loss isn't something people generally talk about. Can you imagine if it were? "Hi, let me rain on your pregnancy parade and tell you what happened to me."

Pregnancy loss is painful to discuss, which often makes it something that goes silently suffered. After my losses, my grandmother shared with me that she suffered a loss of a baby boy when she was three months along. Up until that point, I never even knew she had lived through that experience. Later she went on to have three girls: my mom and two aunts. My point is that I would have never known about my potential would-have-been uncle if she didn't share her story with me after my loss.

I believe there is something to be said for those of us who have suffered a loss or losses on top of having to continue baby-making with infertility. It's an entirely different kind of loss and feeling alone that not everyone understands. Not only do you carry the weight of losing your bun or buns, but you also might be wrestling with the feeling that you might have missed your only chance, or lost the only baby or babies you might ever have. On top of that, pregnancy doesn't come easily to you, and you might also not know how you are going to afford additional treatments.

Hope knows no fault or blame.

People who survive loss know that there comes a time when they have to let the blame go. Kick it to the curb. Escort it to the door. Tell it goodbye and sayonara if they ever hope to make room for hope again. I know what it's like to fall into the trap of thinking that somehow your actions contributed to or caused your loss or losses in part or in full. I blamed myself for years. It didn't matter what my doctors said to contradict my beliefs. I still found a way to assign some of the fault to me.

It's sad that most of us jump to this conclusion, because in almost all cases we couldn't be further from the truth. Real hope knows no fault or blame. It knows that tragedies sometimes happen to even the best parent-to-be.

Feel then forgive.

It's okay to question everything. It's okay to get angry. It's okay to feel all that you feel. Hope comes when you don't stay pissed. When you release blame. When you are ready, forgive yourself. It isn't your fault. Help your mind and your heart become more understanding and forgiving of that fact. You really did everything you could. Believe that. By bullying yourself and choosing to look at only part of the bigger picture, you are only bringing more pain to already overpained you. Pain is the last thing you need more of right now. Blaming yourself won't bring your baby or babies back and will keep you from being able to fully honor your child or children.

On the other hand, forgiving yourself may lead you to believe you are worthy of another chance. Another possibility. Another outcome. Feeling then forgiving is all about getting out all that you wish you had done differently. If you have to, write a letter. I made a memory box for my firstborn sons, and every time I wrote a letter to them I rolled it up, tied it with a bow, and left it for them in their box. It was kind of a mailbox to Heaven sort of thing. Here is one of the letters I wrote.

My dear Ryan and Brayden,

I begged every power in the world to keep you with me but that didn't happen. My heart and belly still can't grasp that we aren't together anymore. I will never ever forget what it felt like holding you in my belly for so long and in my arms for such a short time. I remember every kick, every hiccup and every second spent with you. I remember the warmth that you radiated through every ultrasound, every milestone and when we were almost to our finish line. And I remember the day we were forced to say goodbye.

I came alive when I learned the news that your Dad and I were blessed to finally have you. I lost myself when you left. I'm still trying to make sense of things even though I know there are no real answers. Losing you hurts so very bad. I am sorry for so many things. My list seems to go on forever.

I am sorry that I've been angry and not able to understand why things happened the way they did. Why you couldn't stay, and why I couldn't keep you no matter how hard I tried. I am sorry this happened. I am sorry that I couldn't hold on even harder. I am sorry I couldn't do more to save your life. I am sorry I didn't tell you I love you more times than I did. I always thought I would have the chance to tell you that when you were born. I am sorry there were times that I was so tired from not sleeping that I feel asleep and missed your every move. I tried. I never knew you were going to be gone. I am sorry that instead of smothering you in person with happy tears all that I did was sob. I was trying to take it all in. I couldn't handle you being there and then swept away. I am sorry that this Mother's Day, our first Mother's Day, that we are spending it apart and that you are there and I am here. I am sorry we made it so far and didn't make it at the same time. I am sorry that I got to hold your hands and feet but you couldn't clench mine and feel me holding you tight.

I'm still begging for your peace and that you are in a place where you are loved and safe from pain. I pray that as brothers you are still together and I pray that one day you will return to me or I will return to you. I pray you will always know me as your mom because I will always know you as my boys even if I can't be where you are. I carried you beyond my belly. I carried you (and still carry you) in my soul. You will be a constant reminder in my life to never give up if I am ever given another chance. You are my stars in the sky.

I love you now and forever,

♡ Mom

Keep singing their song.

When I was first admitted to the hospital for preterm premature rupture of membranes with our firstborn sons, my husband downloaded some of my favorite songs onto my MP3 player so that I would have a little something to keep me and the boys company in the hospital. I kept it next to my hospital bed and played it to keep me calm and focused. He knows I like upbeat and optimistic tunes. During the pregnancy and when I was holding onto them for dear life, I sang to them every day. Once they were gone, I didn't know if I would ever sing again.

Their lullabies eventually did find me again. It comes as no surprise, really, because it was the last thing I was doing with them. It was that last moment when I was holding them, when I felt whole and complete. It has been said that babies recognize their mama's voice from the womb. I wondered if mine had time in those five months, going on six, to memorize mine. I hoped they had. As it already was, I couldn't help but keep replaying all that had happened over and over like lyrics in my head. I wanted time to stop so that I could unwind everything that had gone wrong. I wanted them back, but I couldn't get to them. One way I felt that I could still be close to them and that they could still hear me was by singing to them.

You don't have to keep sing the same songs. You can choose new ones. Just keep singing something.

Promise to carry on your bun's life with your life.

It took me what seemed to be an eternity before realizing that the single greatest way for me to honor my three babies was to live out the life that they could not. I spent some time thinking about what type of mom they would want me to be to them if they were somehow here. I tried to imagine that they could somehow see me and hear me and watch me even if I couldn't see them. I also thought about what I would say to them if they asked me to keep living for them. Without even having to think, I knew my answer. It wouldn't be no, I can't. It wouldn't be I don't know how, so I am

169

not going to, or, I am hurting too bad. I knew the answer inside me was, with all that I am, for you, I absolutely will. I might not know how yet, but as your mom, you of course can count on me. I will figure it out.

It's not easy thinking about carrying on your bun's life when it feels as though their life is meant to be lived right here with you. This is the part that no one tells you about. This is the part of some of our journeys that makes having hope so hard. But if you can find a way, the same way I did, I promise that you will see your little buns in everything you do. No, it will never be the same as having them here. But it will be better than the alternative, which is forgetting them and forever keeping them in memory rather than giving them more moments lived.

In order to get myself to the point where I could begin carrying on their lives with my own, I had to begin thinking differently. Basically, I had to contemplate the opposite and play that out in my mind. What if I didn't carry on their lives with mine? What if I just closed off and curled up into a ball and refused to do anything? What then? What if this was all that they could see and remember me by? What would that do to them? What would that do to me? What would it do to their dad, my husband, and what would it do to the marriage we still have left? Is that what they would have wanted?

I knew deep down inside that in order for me to truly honor my little buns lost, I had to return to the parts of myself that I was when they were here. The person I was when I held them. When I was fighting for them. When I wouldn't let go. In some small way I was hoping they could see their mom as a fighter. So that is what I did. I chose to be their fighter. I chose to be their mom. I chose to never leave. That is how I wanted my babies to see me.

When I held my boys before they had to go, I had no power to save them. I promised them silently and in my heart that I would do the best that I could to carry on their life and message to other people. And that's what I set out to do. I wanted to do everything that I could to help prevent any other family from going through what we had gone through. I felt that anything short of that would not serve their purpose in my life.

In wanting to get involved to help make the fight against TTTS even stronger, I went online to the Twin-to-Twin Transfusion Syndrome Foundation and read about how the organization has been compiling information about monochorionic twin and triplet pregnancies since 1995 and uses the information to try to find a link between pregnancies and treatments. That moment I decided I wanted to donate my medical file (my record of their life) to research, hoping that somehow my boys could be a part of a future cure and other mommies' and daddies' hope.

I sent away for the International TTTS Registry packet and completed it. It was sixteen pages long. That might not sound like much, but every page crushed my heart. It came with a personal note from the founder. Instantly I found my very first TTTS mommy friend. Even though I hadn't met her face-to-face, her scribbled note meant the world to me. Here was a mom who devoted her life to a promise kept to her two sons lost to TTTS.

I had to order all of my medical records to send along with it. It was one of the hardest things I have ever done but one of the most rewarding things in the end. I sobbed the entire time I read through all of my medical reports and doctor's notes. The only way I got through the tears was to keep reminding myself that I was doing it to honor my boys, and that my contribution to research might give other future families a fighting chance. Here's a copy of the letter I sent along with the registry packet.

Dear Mary:

Please find our enclosed International TTTS Registry paperwork. Our wish and our prayer is that our information will be used to help further TTTS research, improve detection and successful intervention, and to find a cure so that no family should ever have to suffer the ill effects of TTTS.

Today and always we join the fight to honor our forever boys, Ryan and Brayden, and to honor you and your Matthew and Steven. We are grateful for all of the work you and your foundation do to make a difference.

With love and thanks to you and our TTTS family,

Join a cause that speaks to you.

Every year during TTTS awareness week in December, my husband and I wear our ribbons. We are going to send away for two more. Well, three more, one for Jake's dog collar, too.

Maybe tying yourself to the actual root cause of your bun's passing is just too much to be a part of. There was a time that I didn't think that I would be able to donate my file to research. Once I did, though, I was finally able to stand back, sob in my husband's arms, and give a special little shout-out to my little buns, as I whispered between my tears, "I did this for you."

Close friends of ours, Eric and Michelle, along with their kids, set up a page for our sons as part of the annual March of Dimes Walk For Babies they participate in each year to honor the son and daughter they lost during their family-building. At first I was hesitant to participate because I felt the group was just too general for me, but when their three sons decided to walk on behalf of our boys, it brought the walk closer to me. We made a contribution online, but it felt too soon to get out there and to face the world. I had mixed feelings about actually doing the walk part. I really wanted to, but I identified with the TTTS walk more.

The day of the walk, my husband and I decided that we would at least stop by to cheer our friends on. I took Ryan and Brayden's little hats and pinned them on our shirts. I wrote their names on cards, made necklaces out of them, and we each wore one. We called our friends on their cell phone while they were walking, and they told us the name of the street they had just passed. We pulled up along the side of the road and saw them walking. We honked and my husband and I grasped hands. After our friends passed by with the crowd, my husband and I decided to get back in the car and try to catch up with them farther down the road. We found a parking spot, parked, and joined them for the remaining part of the walk. I was so glad that we did.

I lost it when we crossed the finish line. To make matters even more difficult, a gal running a booth advertising a boot camp for moms who was passing out energy bars attempted to recruit me.

She was bubbly and clueless, and I remember being caught off-guard and wanting to say, "Hello, are you even paying attention? Some of us don't have our babies here." We had our firstborn sons' official TTTS awareness ribbons on along with the number of weeks of gestation when they passed away written on our shirts. She obviously wasn't paying attention. It was hard to forgive such an oversight at first. But later, I let it go. She was just one small blip in that day. I was reminded by my husband that it is a good thing that some people don't know what to say, because if they did, it would mean that they have been through something similar, something we wouldn't wish on anyone.

Build hope filled memories.

There are always going to be painful reminders. The best way to bring hope back into your baby-making is to also have hopeful ones.

Since that first walk, the March of Dimes has become part of our family. The following year I participated in the their family quilt project while my husband and friends walked on our sons' behalf as I was on bed rest. All of the families who lost a baby were given a fabric square to decorate. In the end, all of the squares were tied together to make into quilts. I thought of it as my boys' baby blanket that I never got to give them. To me it represented a sort of baby blanket to send up to Heaven type of thing.

Prior to this, the only thing I have ever sewn is a button, but I was determined to make the most beautiful baby blanket I could. I bought some fabric that had a kangaroo on it with a baby kangaroo in her pouch. The lady at the cash register asked me what I was doing. Tears were streaming down my cheeks as I told her I was making a baby blanket for my babies that passed away and that I wanted the mommy kangaroo to represent me.

It took me awhile to sew the whole thing by hand, but little by little my vision came together. I cut out a second baby kangaroo and lined it up just right so that it looked like the kangaroo had twin baby kangaroos. I bought two pairs of little combat boot buttons, two miniature metal dog tags that said "little trooper" on them, and a button that said "courage and honor" on it along with two plastic pins that said "hero" on them. I sewed the elements on the blanket. I cried every time I added something new. I fastened two TTTS awareness ribbons to the blanket as well. I made the giraffe represent my husband and turtle represent our dog Jake. I wanted our boys to feel surrounded by the family that loves them. I sewed an elephant on it to represent the popular saying that elephants never forget.

When the blanket was finally finished, I cried all over again. It was hard to give it up, but at the same time it wasn't. It was their blanket now and it no longer belonged to me. It became part of something bigger. Later that year, my husband contacted the March of Dimes. They have always been so good to us. He said, "I know this sounds like a crazy request, but my wife wasn't able to participate in the walk and never really got to see her quilt because of all that we have been going through to build our family." Within a few days, one of their family team specialists tracked it down and emailed us picture of it. I couldn't believe my eyes. It meant so much to me.

Around this same time, I began turning our garden into a memory garden, a place where my hope for my future could bloom. On a tight budget, I chose small simple things that could still make a big impact. To honor my little buns lost, I placed three small wrought-iron bird garden accents and perched them above our front door. To bring the soothing sound of water, I bought a wall-mounted fountain and hung it on the wall closest to the window so that I could hear it even when I was inside. At night the fountain lights up, illuminating the dark, a little something to help me find my way when it's hard to see. I planted two kangaroo paw plants along the picket fence. They produce beautiful, velvety flowers on long stems, something I could actually nurture and watch grow.

The kangaroo paw flower is remarkably like the paw of the kangaroo. As a once mommy to babies that I carried and were with me, I identify with a kangaroo mommy who carries her young in her pouch. Kangaroos can have up to three babies at a time. When one baby, also known as a joey, becomes mature and is just out of the pouch, another can be developing in the pouch while one embryo is in a pause mode. I planted the kangaroo paws to remind me that hope repeats itself.

Carry them with you.

I knew right away that I wanted (and achingly needed) something to hold onto to give me a way of carrying them with me. It took me awhile to figure out just what that could be. I decided on a necklace. My husband bought me a necklace with two initials. One R. One B.

For my fortieth birthday my family wanted to all pitch in to get me something special. They asked me what I wanted. I told them that I wanted something to represent all of my little guys. I first found a necklace that I liked with the birthstones of both my firstborn and second born sons, but there was a mix-up on the site, and even though it was listed as in stock, it actually wasn't. No more like it were going to be made. I am not really a materialistic person, and I usually don't get sad over material things, but I remember feeling sad. Here I had chosen the perfect necklace. I was stuck on the necklace for a couple of days. I kept thinking about it. But the necklace wasn't to be. I ended up choosing a ring set, made by the same designer. There are three rings total that meet up with a central round green amethyst stone. This would have been my firstborn little guys' birthstone. I chose it to represent them.

It is said that the green amethyst is the stone of harmony. Being a musical gal, that is how I relate to the world and that is how I feel being bonded to my children. Like all the musical notes come together and give my life a meaningful song. The outer two rings are smooth solid sterling silver bands. I chose them to represent my two little guys now. They have me wrapped around their fingers. The pastel green amethyst solitaire is soft like a baby nursery. It is reflective. It is tranquil and hopeful to look at. It reminds me of an infinity pool and to me, it represents my love for my babies extending to infinity. Being round it reminds me of my belly and represents my hope coming full circle. I wear the rings all of the time. Besides my wedding band and engagement ring, they are the only other rings I ever wear. The cost of the ring set was fairly affordable. It was $155.

To make Father's Day a better memory for my husband, I purchased a set of stainless steel dog tags, had them engraved, and gave them to him on his first Father's Day after our boys passed away. One of the tags reads "Forever An Amazing Dad." The other reads "Ryan & Brayden Our Forever Boys." My husband has been known for carrying them in his pocket, taking them to work and on trips. I have been known to sleep with them under my pillow and wear them around my neck.

The day our Brecken and Caden were born, my husband surprised me by taking them out of the pocket of his scrubs and showing them to me. I was still speechless over everything else going on. Being back in the same operating room. We even ended up in the exact same recovery room. A sign to me that our firstborn sons were with us.

Be someone's hope angel.

My husband mentioned to me that one of his buddies and his buddy's wife were struggling with trying to get pregnant and were considering a consultation at the fertility clinic we had gone to but were filled with questions. My husband got back in touch with him with an email I put together offering to share our knowledge and experiences if they were interested. In the email, I told him a little bit about the practice and to tell his wife that she's in good hands and that we've been in a similar place. I wrote that I've also been pretty private with the fertility stuff, and it certainly isn't any easier living where we live with kids and strollers everywhere we look. I went on to say that at first the process can be a little overwhelming, but that they will likely get into a routine and it is manageable. I added that my husband and I would be there for them however we could help or to answer any of their questions.

My husband's friend and his wife took us up on our invitation and met us at our home not too long after that. We had just had our boys, and knowing that it might be tough for her to sit with us while our newborns slept, I made her a gift and placed it in a natural-colored jute bag with a little bird and bee on it. It was something to represent the baby-making that she had ahead of her. It was something to take the focus off of us in that moment, so that we could just focus on her and the two of them.

In this capacity, I was finally able to give a little something back and be like the couple that our friends Erin and Brian were to us. In the hope bag was a miniature hope book, a little bird's nest with a bag of tiny eggs to put in the nest after she had her egg retrieval, a miniature wishing well bucket, a tiny compass, and a small pair of plastic combat boots. Attached to the nest and bag of eggs were two small sterling silver charms that I bought at the craft store. One of the charms had the word "Destiny" written on it. The other charm had the word "Family." Inside the hope book were individual pages that read: "Our Story," "Time Together," "In the moment," "Just Believe," "Someday," "Right Before My Eyes," "Peace," and "Our Family." I left the last few pages blank and told her she would some-day write her own happy ending, or beginning really.

I choked up when it came time to tell her the story behind the compass and what it was intended to be. With her husband sitting right beside her I looked at them and then I told her, "This is for you if you ever lose your way. At one point I lost mine, and it was really hard for me to find my way back. If I had a compass like this, it probably would have helped because it would have reminded me of where I was headed. Remember to love one another through every minute." She thanked me. We hugged and they left.

My heart danced when I learned that their daughter was con-ceived via IVF their very next cycle. I never thought I would be able to give someone else hope. My little buns lost and my newfound buns all gave me the strength to do that. I look forward to getting to be a part of their daughter's life and watching her grow up. I remember when she was just a tiny hope seed in her mommy and daddy's heart while they were sitting on my sofa.

Let someone be your hope angel.

I am one of those people who is much better at giving than taking, so letting someone be my angel wasn't something I necessarily knew how to do or was good at. Lucky for me, my newfound angel found me and led the way.

Right after we lost our firstborn sons, a new family moved in two doors down from us. When they introduced one of their four sons to me, my mouth dropped and my heart sank. "This is Brayden," they said. At first I didn't know how to take it or how to respond. One of our sons who passed away we named Brayden. I admit I was dazed and sadness filled me. They probably saw it in my face. Even with all that I was feeling, I shook his little, four-year-old hand. I could have just stood there and held onto it forever, but I shook it for the appropriate length of time and then let go.

I remember silently questioning how I was going to be able to do this. How was I going to be able to hear my son's name on a regular basis assigned to another little boy? I wondered how this could have happened. I mean, what are the odds, and how very cruel of life it seemed. How could I see his little smile without thinking of our boys.

The first couple of days I heard his name over and over through our windows, and I seriously contemplated the thought of moving. I was still heartbroken and I was torn. I came to realize that if we were going to stay in the neighborhood that I would have to find peace with it somehow. I didn't know it yet, but my new little neighbor would eventually become my hope angel.

It took me a little while, but Brayden made it easy. He was always waving, smiling, and approaching me every time I was out on the patio watering our plants or out on the front lawn with our dog Jake. No matter where I was, there he was—playing, laughing, but always including me. At times he would even yell my name from the car window. I remember one day telling my husband,

"You know, in a way it's kind of neat. Here we get to see a little boy, with our son's name, live and grow next to us." We get to watch another Brayden grow up in our neighborhood and we will always look at him in kind of a special way because he shares a bond, without even knowing it, with our son. It's only a name bond, but it is a bond nevertheless.

Our neighbor Brayden is eight now. He's finally at that age where he's just old enough to start helping my husband and I with our boys. When my husband is away Brayden helps out a couple of days a week, and watches over the boys when they are out in the front of the house with me riding around on their swivel cars. Brayden does a great job making sure that they ride safely, that their helmets stay on, and he's especially good at helping to coach my boys to stay within the set boundaries.

Not only am I blessed to be able to watch Brayden grow up, but seeing the joy on my boys faces when they interact with him and how they both look up to him absolutely melts my heart beyond words.

The other day just reinforced for me, once again, that Brayden truly is my hope angel. At the end of his babysitting session he brought the boy's swivel cars back to the front of our house and stood outside our fence as the boys and I said our goodbyes. Then he did something that I've never seen him to. He reached into his pocket. Before showing me anything he shared with me that in his classroom at school they had been making torn paper art, also known as tear art. He then pulled out a folded orange piece of paper with beautifully torn edges. He said, "I made one for you and one for my mom. It's a pumpkin that looks like a heart." He unfolded it and placed it in my hand. I hardly had words. It reminded me of that same speechless moment I had the first time I shook his hand four years ago. I thanked him for such a thoughtful gift and told him that it had a new home on the front on my refrigerator door.

From that point on, the fall season has never been the same. Every time I see a pumpkin, my heart beams like the northern lights.

Opening up my pained heart to one small kiddo and his daily small acts of kindness was singlehandedly the most healing thing I've ever done. I'm pretty certain that Brayden never sees me wipe my tears of gratefulness when he leaves, but I do every time he leaves our front porch.

When you're ready, find your Brayden, or let your Brayden find you.

Leave yourself a hope after loss note.

If it helps, write yourself your own special kind of hope note. Your hope-after-loss hope note. I asked my husband to write one for me in our treatment journal that I keep. It meant a lot having a note that came from him. He wrote it the day we were given the green light by our reproductive endocrinologist to begin our next cycle. Here's what his note said:

"Yay! Dr. Anderson gave us the ok to start on Saturday. Given everything that has happened, we are really blessed to be healthy and have this opportunity again. It will be once again a real tough experience for Sandi, but my wife is amazingly strong and resilient and the day will come that Ryan and Brayden will have a sibling. I deeply love you all for everything that you have endured and given to this family."

On days when I had hope note writer's block, I would simply keep hope texts and hope notes that I received from others nearby. One particular note that stands out to me is one given to me by the mother of a friend. She and I met only once. It was during Thanksgiving. I will never forget her. We briefly talked about what happened. I don't know how it came up, she is just one of those people who instantly gets it. She suffered a loss, too. I don't re-member much about our conversation, but talking to her was like talking to my mom. Being in different places during the holidays I just really missed my own mom. At that moment I needed an older, wiser mommy owl to comfort me, and that's what she was.

At Christmas, out of nowhere she sent me a gift and a greeting card. I was so surprised to get a gift from someone I felt I hardly knew. With it was a note that read:

"Dear Sandi, I was so touched by you and enjoyed meeting you! Wanted to give you a hat and scarf. Wrap it around your neck twice. I wish you a healthy and happy new year. All the best. Love, P."

I remember thinking, wow. She made this for me? Wrap it around your neck twice? Aw. Was that her way of telling me that my two will always be with me? I kept her note and mailed her a thank-you. I received this reply card back from her:

"Dear Sandi, Your note touched me so much. I have thought of you often. I felt your pain and I also felt you are a strong person. I got a puppy two months ago and it has turned out to be a full time job! I love her but lots of work. Take care and hope to hear from you soon. Love in friendship, P."

While a hope note or two might not seem like much, when you begin collecting the hope notes you do have, your hope can only grow.

When you're ready, troubleshoot, try again, and take another risk.

Your hope is not meant to leave you. If you feel that it has because of all that you have suffered, you will find it again when you are ready. Trying again is hard. Just remember that no step you take is for nothing. It's all for something, even if it doesn't feel that way. Every single step will lead you to your eventual family. Every pregnancy is entirely different, and just because one ends doesn't mean your next one will. Think hope.

Honor your forever mommyness.

There is no second-guessing what I am about to tell you. You are a forever mommy. A forever mommy is someone who is a mom to a little one who has gone on a step ahead. In this case, she's you. The world doesn't necessarily get to see this part of you or know you in this way. But you know it. I know it. Your baby or babies know it. It is something that can never be taken away from you. Not ever.

One of the hardest questions I still face, even after the birth of my second born sons, is "Are they your first?" Before I tell you what I tell them, thanks for allowing me a courtesy rant for a second. Even though it's harmless, why do people always ask that? I never ask that question. Do you? I think anyone who has faced baby-making difficulties probably never asks that question. Just like we probably don't go around asking people if they have any kids yet. Regardless, at some point, you too will probably be asked the question. Sometimes I answer no. Sometimes I respond yes. It all depends on who's asking. Not because I don't want to answer or don't know how to answer, but because I reserve my real answer, my real truth, my forever mommyness, for the people I think will understand. I reserve it for people like you.

Find a forever mommy friend.

We forever mommies need each other. Even when we don't know one another personally, we still huddle together nonetheless. We share pain and we talk to each other in our own kind of forever mommy signals. We silently "get it" and "get each other," even if our paths never cross.

It doesn't take the pain away, but it sure helps having a friend who acknowledges and remembers your little one's life. In fact one of my forever mommy friends lost her daughter in a different year but in the same month that I lost my firstborn boys. The anniversary of her daughter's passing and my firstborn sons' passing is just five days apart.

We don't talk as often as I'd like to right now, just because of our differing schedules and kiddos' stages, but we both have each other's angels on our minds. Last week, in response to the message she posted to her daughter, I wrote on her Facebook wall, "She will always know you as her forever mommy." Today, she wrote on my wall, "Your boys are with you always." She also put a frowny face and a smiley face at the same time.

If you haven't made another forever mommy friend yet, consider me your first. The forever mommy in me honors, hugs, and hopes for the forever mommy in you. As forever mommies go, we are all connected. To deny your forever mommy title is to deny everyone else's. Forever mommies know that it's not about moving on. It's about always remembering.

Notice hope.

We all want our baby-making to be simple. But infertility sometimes makes it terribly complex. But as tangled as it gets, there is always hope to be found, noticed, and invited back.

Sometime in the midst of all that I was going through, my dad sent me a book. With it was a note: "Thought you'd like to read this. Love, Dad." It was Dean Koontz's A Big Little Life: A Memoir of a Joyful Dog. He knows how much I love my Jakey dog. He also knows how to say a lot without saying much at all. I didn't read it right away. I couldn't bear the thought of anymore loss, of any kind, especially the thought of losing my own dog. In a nutshell, it was just too much for me at the time, so I kept it in my nightstand with the intention of picking it up when I was ready.

When I eventually did pick up the book, it seemed it found me at that exact time and place for a reason. The book touches on love and loss and how little lives, like every life, can change the lives of others. It maintains that no life is small and that every life is big. Reading Trixie's memoir did in fact make me cry. But woven in those pages emerged a message of hope so strong that I couldn't help but wonder if it was meant just for me. If a certain series of events hadn't lined up the way they did for Dean and his wife, they would have ended up with a different dog, and their life would not have been the same. I couldn't help but think of the striking parallels between the author's story and my own, about how our dogs came into our lives. Amazingly, a book that didn't even have to do with baby-making made me notice something about my baby-making journey I had never noticed before. That is, the story about how all my babies came to me, including how my first baby, my Australian Shepherd named Jake, came to me. First loss. Then hope.

In thinking back to how our Jakey came to us, my husband and I were actually set to get a different dog. A different Australian Shepherd. But just prior to us receiving our soon-to-be puppy, the breeder, Teresa, contacted us and delivered the sad news that, the mother, Teaz, delivered the puppies prematurely. One of the placentas detached and one puppy died. This caused some of the other puppies to become toxic, which caused early labor. Only three puppies made it through. Teresa shared with us that she was devastated by the loss, since Teaz's other litters were so strong and healthy. She told us that unfortunately she only had one black tri (the kind we wanted). It was a male. The five others that were lost were all black tris. Australian Shepherds come in different color variations. A black tri is tricolored. It is black, with tan and white markings.

In an update, Teresa notified us of another loss. One of the girls passed away, but the black tri boy and the other blue merle girl were hanging in there. A blue merle's markings are marbled black, white and gray. She said she was starting to have hope that they would make it. The two surviving pups were being tube-fed every four hours to get their strength up. She said she was thinking of calling them Rocky and Laila (Ali) because they had to fight so hard. I emailed Teresa back right away that my husband and I would absolutely welcome a little trooper like Rocky into our home. I began saying prayers for them and began preparing myself to be Rocky's mommy. The next day, Teresa wrote me this message:

Sandi,

It breaks my heart to have to tell you that we lost Rocky last night. He was smaller and weaker than Laila but the fact that he had made it this far gave us hope that he would survive. I have to believe that his life would not have been a quality one and that this outcome was best for him so that he is not suffering. He fought so hard. Your offer to give him a loving home was so wonderful. You and your husband are exactly the kind of people we want our puppies to go to. I wish things had been different. We hope that Laila will survive, it is just unbelievable that we only have one puppy left. I wish that I had better news, but as I said before we will do whatever we can to help you find a puppy. I know of one litter that is 3 weeks old and there are several tris, if you are interested let me know. I'll keep you posted on Laila's progress. We've decided that if she survives she will be staying with us, we've been through too much with her at this point to let her go.

— Teresa

The next day, New Year's Day, followed Teresa's next email. Once again she had bad news to pass along to us. She explained in her email that Laila passed away the night before, and she guessed the litter was just not meant to be and that she didn't understand why it had to happen. She said that Teaz looked for her puppies but seemed to have accepted that they were gone. She went on to say we would be great owners and she knew the right puppy was out there waiting for us, and thanked us for our support. I remember crying not only for our lost puppy-to-be but also for Teaz. The thought of any mommy being without her babies makes my heart hurt.

In my response to Teresa, I signed off, "Kiss Teaz for us." I remember feeling so sad and so very empty. I didn't understand how something like this could happen. How did I go from being a doggy mommy anxiously awaiting my little puppy to not having one at all? Little did I know I would later go on and relate to Teaz in a way that I had never imagined. Like Teaz, I had a healthy, strong pregnancy with my first twin pregnancy. Then sudden complications. Then preterm labor. Then loss of one due to infection. Then loss of two due to the complications with my first one. Then endless searching for my lost litter. It was hard for me to accept that they were gone.

Hope ended up coming full circle for me, and I wish the same had been true for Teaz. Teresa informed us that the litter that we were interested in was actually Teaz's fourth. In her first litter, born in 2000, she had two males. Her son, Willie, was part of the breeder's lives until they lost him to cancer a couple of years ago. Teaz's second litter was born in 2002 and consisted of seven puppies. Her third litter, again seven puppies, was born in 2005. Rocky and Laila were her final litter and after everything she went through the breeder chose not to breed her again. They lost Teaz in 2011. She died in her sleep at the age of thirteen. Teaz's kids Zap, Flirt and Gader and grandkids Abby and Karma carry on her spirit.

My husband and I knew that we would never be able to replace our little fighter Rocky, the little pup we loved from afar but never got to meet, but our hearts were still set on getting a puppy. A puppy was going to mark the start of our family, and we wanted to raise one as our own, together. My husband contacted another breeder that had a new litter and surprised me with the news. We were going to go pick one out. When we arrived at the breeder's house, I felt like a little kid. I was so excited I could hardly stand still. She brought us to the puppies. The sight was irresistible. I would have taken all of them if we could have. I was instantly attached.

One of the baby blue merle puppies wrapped itself around my husband's arm and just held on. It wouldn't let go, and both of our hearts just melted. The rush of holding our potential first baby together was something I will never forget. We had wanted a black tri all along, but this little guy was tugging at our hearts. There was something special about him. Usually blue merles have blue eyes; this puppy's eyes were both brown. He was adorable, and as far as I could tell, my husband and I were on the same page. We were set on him.

It would be some time before he could come home with us because he was still too little, so we had to say our goodbyes for now. I remember feeling like we finally had the puppy we had always dreamed of. As we were wrapping up our tour, we passed through the backyard. The breeder's entire backyard was filled with kennels and play areas and older dogs. There were a few dogs staring at us through a gate. Being an Australian Shepherd lover, I could hardly resist the sight of all of them. I asked the breeder if I could go say hello.

The breeder opened the gate and a one-year-old black tri male came right up to us. He ran right past the food being dished out for chow time. We both kneeled to pet him. He rolled onto his back as if to gesture for us to rub his belly and so we did. Then he burped in our face. My husband and I laughed. It felt as if he had been our dog the entire time. I kept thinking of the puppy that my husband just cuddled, but I couldn't shake the feeling of Jake.

It was tough passing up the cute puppy, but we ended up choosing Jake. Well, Jake chose us. Since then, our lives have never been the same. Without even knowing it, it seemed all along that Jake was destined to be our pup. I had no idea that my boys, Brecken and Caden, would also come to me in a similar way that Jake did. First would come loss. Then would come hope. Then would come a life filled with joy and motherhood in every imaginable way.

I still get teary-eyed thinking about Teaz. Without ever meeting her in person she still had such a big impact on my life. She brought my dog into my life that I might not have known otherwise. In a recent email, Teresa updated me that she will be breeding Teaz's beautiful granddaughter Karma in 2013 and that she is looking forward to seeing Teaz's sweet personality in her great grandchildren.

Trixie's doggy memoir brought me back to where all of my hope to become a mommy first started. It started with Teaz. When I finished reading the final pages, I couldn't get the title out of my head. A big little life. Wow, was that certainly appropriate. Not only was I reminded of Jake and how he helped me to survive all of my pain. I was reminded of firstborn sons' lives. Their lives were little and at the same time they were also big. They were little because their bodies were small and their lives were cut short. They were big because they led me to my destiny. Their amazing two brothers.

Decide where your hope will take you.

I allow myself to smile now. I have to be strong for my Brecken and Caden. They are my troopers of all troopers who endured it all with me. They are my hope after loss. It is the passing of my first puppy that led to my Jake. And it is the passing of my first three buns that led me to questions that later became answers, that later became preventative treatment, which ultimately led me to trying to again, which is every reason why I am where I am today. The hope I carried for all of them and still carry with me gives me the strength to talk about their tragedy.

The hope we hold for our little ones that we lose needs to go somewhere. If you close it out and shut it down, it only diminishes their memory A few days ago actually marked the three-year anniversary of Ryan and Brayden's passing. I can't believe it has been three years. It's almost fitting that I am completing this book around the same time. My love and my hope for them never fades. They continue to be a part of everything hopeful I ever do.

What will you do with the hope you carried and still carry in your heart and memory, forever mama? Will you use it to help you heal? Will you use to help you try again? Will you use it to consider donor eggs or donor sperm? Will you use it to explore adoption if that is where you decide to go? Your hope knows no limits. Where will you let your hope for your buns, both "passed" (not past, because they are always a part of you) and future, take you?

inspire your hopeful future

IT'S TIME TO make room for that hopeful future of yours that lies ahead and awaits you. If after reading all of these pages a small part of you is still doubting your future and wondering why you just can't just wing it without hope, I will tell you.

When you have hope you're able to see your way out of it. You make a better baby-maker. You carry the bigger picture in your mind. You gain the mindset that you can succeed. You lessen some of the stressors. You're able to work hard for something that you know will come. You're open to opportunities. You close no doors. You stop doubting. What's more, you stop second-guessing. You free your mind. You're able to steer when the road is wobbly. You have more fight in you for the fight itself, and less fight in you toward yourself. You add a little happy to your miserable. You make decisions that will be the right ones. You'll be able to see for yourself why all of it is worth it.

Your hope is not meant to be stored away and saved up for only your more promising baby-making moments. There is no "I will hope tomorrow." Let yourself hope right now. One hope step at a time. It is the best baby-making friend you will ever make. It is also the greatest gift you will ever keep, because when you eventually do have that family of yours—and you will, it's just a matter of time—you'll be able to teach it to your child or children. The life lesson of what it means to believe in yourself and commit to your path. In turn, they will be able to follow their hope all of their lives as they pursue their goals and navigate through life's tougher times.

And when that day comes, when they ask you where did I come from? You can tell them that it was hope that led you to where they are. It kept you trying for them even when it seemed there was no hope all.

from my oven to yours

Dear Bunless Buddy,

This letter is for the you ahead of you. The you who will make it through to the other side where you will have the family you have worked so hard for. The you who will finally be a mom.

Before you get there, I wish I could say that this will be easy for you, but it might not be. At times you might struggle. You might even want to hide from yourself and the rest of the world when the pain starts to run too deep and hurt too bad. I wish I could say there will be no tears, but there might be rivers along the way. In fact, you will probably never cry so hard in all your life. But each tear will bring you to take another step.

You might even lose some battles before you actually win any. None of them will be your fault. Pushing through the pain of it all might take a lot. You might not think you can do it, but you can. You will eventually win, and when you do, you will understand why it was all worth it.

There are probably going to be times when you are going to think that the Universe must not like you or that you did something wrong to be going seemingly nowhere while the rest of the world seems to reach their somewhere over the rainbow. But your circles will turn into roads and lead you to the place you dream of, and you will end up right where you want to be. Your little one or little ones will have your resilience and tenacity.

At times it will be hard for a part of you to believe that they are actually here for real. You might even have to keep pinching yourself to believe it. You used to wonder if your life was going to be empty forever. Now you know it's not. You will have joy and love in your life like you have never known.

Just remember, fight hard, recharge often, and don't let your infertility stand in your way. Forgive yourself for feeling over-whelmed. Once you find hope, hold onto it and don't let go. Your hope will the lead the way.

Most importantly, never give up no matter how hopeless every-thing seems. It might take longer than you planned, but you will get there, you will make it, and you will see you soon!

Your friend always,

♡ Sandi

P.S. Even though someday your hair might be a mess, your toes might not be painted, and the only thing you thing you might have eaten so far today is a piece of your kiddo's English muffin with peanut butter and honey, you are happier than you've ever been.